BRAIN IMAGING *in*
SCHIZOPHRENIA

Insights and Applications

Published by ReMEDICA Publishing Limited
32-38 Osnaburgh Street, London, NW1 3ND, UK

Tel: +44 207 388 7677
Fax: +44 207 388 7678
Email: books@remedica.com
www.remedica.com

© 2000 ReMEDICA Publishing Limited
Publication date November 2000

ISBN 1 901346 08 0

British Library Cataloguing-in-Publication Data
A catalogue record for this book is available from the British Library.

BRAIN IMAGING *in* SCHIZOPHRENIA

Insights and Applications

TONMOY SHARMA
XAVIER CHITNIS

Institute of Psychiatry
London, UK

ReMEDICAPUBLISHING

Contents

Introduction

The application of brain imaging to the study of psychiatric disorders has revolutionized research into the biological basis of schizophrenia. In vivo imaging techniques have allowed researchers to identify changes in brain structure and function, and to examine their relationships with medication, genetics, clinical profile and cognitive functioning. Brain imaging provides contemporary psychiatry with graphical insights into the pathophysiology of schizophrenia, and objective methods for studying the underlying neurobiology of the disorder.

The history of brain imaging in schizophrenia is relatively brief and the field continues to grow rapidly. Until the late 1970s, studies of brain structure in psychiatric disorders were mainly limited to post-mortem work, greatly limiting the range of clinical populations that could be studied. With the advent of computed tomography (CT) scanning, and the later move to magnetic resonance imaging (MRI), it has become possible to undertake longitudinal studies, and to examine, at a minute level, brain structures that may be important in the pathogenesis of schizophrenia. Research is now beginning to examine the temporal incidence of structural changes, and how they may reflect the expression of genetic liability to the illness.

Functional imaging methodologies such as positron emission tomography (PET) and single photon emission computed tomography (SPECT) allow us to study cerebral blood flow, neurotransmitter receptor number and function, and regional metabolic activity. At an even more advanced level of investigation, functional MRI (fMRI) exploits the close association between neuronal synaptic activity, energy metabolism and blood circulation, to yield sophisticated images of functional activity of specific brain regions. Magnetic resonance spectroscopy (MRS) is a technique that is used to measure the regional levels of chemical compounds, facilitating the in vivo study of neurochemistry. Studies of schizophrenia using these methods have demonstrated widespread changes in brain activity, at both a chemical and vascular level.

This text provides an overview of the major techniques used in psychiatric neuroimaging, together with a summary of findings from their applications to schizophrenia research. Chapters 1 and 2 outline the major structural and functional imaging techniques, explaining the basic principles together with their applications, contraindications, relative merits and limitations. Representative images are also provided. Chapters 3 and 4 illustrate how these techniques have been used in schizophrenia research and detail the major findings to date. These chapters attempt to make these findings relevant in terms of clinical practice while also providing an insight into the major theories guiding current research. Chapter 5 examines the influence of genes on brain structure and function, and how this is increasing our understanding of the aetiology of schizophrenia.

Brain Imaging in Schizophrenia

Acknowledgements
We are indebted to all those who provided images for inclusion in this book: Vivienne Curtis, Garry Honey, Ivo Dinov, Shitij Kapur, Anne Lingford-Hughes, Michael Mega, Katherine Narr, Paul Thompson, Mike Travis and Ian Wright.

We wish to acknowledge the contribution of Joanna Kilcooley to the preparation of this text, and we are also very grateful to Ian Wright, Garry Honey and Simon Meara for commenting on early drafts.

CHAPTER 1
Structural Brain Imaging

Computed tomography

Computed tomography (CT) is a rapid, cheap and widely available imaging technique that was introduced into clinical use in the 1970s for studying the anatomy of the brain in vivo. Its introduction transformed the diagnosis and treatment of people with neurological disorders, and re-ignited interest in the biological basis of psychiatric disorders (Table 1).

Early generation scanners consisted of a radiographic tube (the source) that rotated around the subject, pausing at intervals to emit beams of X-rays, whilst an array of synchronously rotating detectors positioned on the opposite side of the body measured the X-rays transmitted through the body. Newer generation machines such as spiral CT scanners consist of multiple constantly rotating X-ray sources, with the signal measured by stationary detectors, and produce higher-resolution images with a shorter scan time.

Table 1. Applications of CT in psychiatry and contraindications for the technique.

Applications in psychiatry	Contraindications
Exclusion of structural disease in patients presenting with possible psychiatric disorder, such as unexplained confusion, movement disorders, psychosis and dementia	Known allergic or anaphylactic reaction to iodine-based contrast media, if needed
Follow-up of abnormal neurological or mental status examinations	In situations where intravenous procedures cannot be used, if needed
In cases where magnetic resonance imaging is contraindicated	Where visualization of subcortical structures may be needed

Principles of CT

CT works on the principle that an image of internal anatomy can be produced by measuring the degree of attenuation of X-rays as they pass through the body (Figure 1). X-rays lose some or all of their energy by interactions with electrons. The degree of attenuation is dependent on both the density of electrons in tissue and the actual tissue density: very few X-rays are able to pass through bone; cerebral tissue is less attenuating; and cerebrospinal fluid (CSF) permits the greatest transmission of X-rays.

Computer algorithms measure the signal intensity recorded by the detectors, and calculate the degree of attenuation at each voxel — literally 'volume pixel' — to form tomographic images of the brain (Figure 2).

CT can distinguish between skull, brain tissue and CSF, but provides relatively poor grey/white matter contrast.

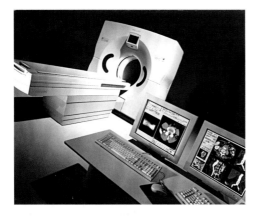

Figure 1. CT scanner.
(Courtesy of Philips Medical Systems.)

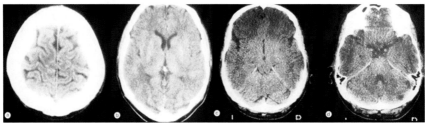

Figure 2. CT brain scans revealing structural detail of the brain surface and ventricles.

CT can also be used to study the cerebral vasculature (CT angiography). Intravenous contrast media such as iodine, which absorbs many more X-rays, is often used to improve the image contrast between blood vessels and surrounding cerebral tissue.

CT scanning is still commonly used in hospital practice, given its relatively low cost and short scan times (Table 2), obviously important in terms of patient comfort. However, brain imaging research has increasingly moved to the use of magnetic resonance imaging (MRI).

Magnetic resonance imaging

Magnetic resonance imaging — or nuclear magnetic resonance imaging as it was originally described — is a non-invasive volume-imaging technology. MRI was introduced as a clinical research tool in the mid-1980s, and its growing popularity and success are attributed to its non-invasive nature, the lack of known risks from magnetic

Table 2. Advantages and limitations of CT imaging.

Advantages	Limitations
Faster, less expensive and more widely available than MRI	Involves the use of X-rays, and hence radiation exposure
Distinguishes between CSF and brain tissue	Intravenous contrast media may be required
Demonstrates the size of ventricles and cerebral sulci	Temporal lobe and subcortical grey matter structures are difficult to visualize

fields and the considerable contrast demonstrated for cerebral tissue (Table 3). MRI presents high-resolution images and has thus come to be recognized as the reference standard in vivo technique for sophisticated exploration of brain anatomy.

Although more expensive than CT, MRI is becoming increasingly widely available in clinical settings. An MRI scan can quickly exclude structural causes in patients presenting with possible neurological or psychiatric problems. Technical advances are even beginning to allow it to be used in image-guided neurosurgery.

Table 3. Applications of MRI in psychiatry and contraindications for the technique.

Applications in psychiatry	Contraindications
Exclusion of stroke, neurological disorder or head injury as causes of symptoms such as confusion, cognitive decline, depression, psychosis, or abnormal neurological signs	Biomedical implants with ferromagnetic properties including defibrillators, neural stimulators, infusion pumps, cochlear implants, aneurysm clips, metallic aortic stents, plates and prostheses
	Pacemakers or a history of invasive heart surgery
	Pregnancy, particularly during the first trimester
	Previous operations to the head, neck or spinal area

Principles of MRI
The magnetic resonance signal is derived from the behaviour of hydrogen atoms in the presence of an external magnetic field, and MRI is made possible by the abundance of water in the human body.

Hydrogen atoms (protons) have a small dipolar magnetic field (they have a north and a south pole), and hence they have an angular momentum — a property known as a spin or magnetic moment, which is often described as being analogous to the motion of a spinning top, or the rotation of the earth around its axis. Normally, the spins of protons are randomly oriented. However, when a person is placed in an MRI scanner, the protons become aligned either parallel or antiparallel to the axis of the magnet. A slightly larger number align themselves parallel, leading to a net magnetization parallel to the axis of the magnet.

The movement of protons around the axis of a magnetic field is called *precession*. The frequency with which they precess about the axis is known as their resonant or *Larmor* frequency, and this is the same for all protons in water. It is important to note that while precessing at the same frequency in a magnetic field, protons may be at different points in their orbit round the axis, and are said not to be precessing *in phase*. Application of a radio-frequency (RF) energy pulse at the exact resonant frequency of protons excites them and disturbs their alignment away from that of the external magnetic field. The amount by which proton spins are shifted from their original alignment is referred to as the flip angle. For example, a 90° flip angle refers to a pulse with sufficient energy to flip the spin orientation into the transverse plane; i.e. they become aligned perpendicular to the external magnetic field (the scanner magnet). The effect of flipping the alignment of the spins is to change the net magnetization to perpendicular to the longitudinal axis of the external field (in the case of a 90° pulse), and to force the protons to precess in phase.

After the RF pulse is turned off and the behaviour of protons is once again determined by the external magnetic field, two processes simultaneously occur. Firstly, in a process known as T_1 relaxation, longitudinal magnetization increases, as proton spins realign themselves parallel to the external magnetic field. T_1, or *spin-lattice* relaxation as it is known, involves protons releasing the energy that was absorbed during the RF pulse by transferring it to local tissue. Secondly, as the spins realign parallel to the external magnet axis, they lose their previous coherent precession, and are said to *dephase*, a process called T_2 decay. The loss of transverse magnetization in T_2 decay is due to the exchange of magnetization between protons as they begin to dephase, and is also called *spin-spin* relaxation. During these processes, the nuclei emit a radiofrequency signal (the MRI signal), which is detected via a receiver coil placed around the patient's head.

There are three types of tissue contrast that can be used in MR scanning. The rates of longitudinal (T_1) and transverse (T_2) relaxation are affected by the local chemical environment, and so it is possible to use T_1 and T_2 relaxation times to differentiate between tissue types in the brain. Similarly, it is possible to distinguish tissue types on the basis of the density of protons. By altering parameters of the scan sequence such as echo time (TE — the time between application of the first pulse of a sequence and MR signal read-out) and repetition time (TR — the time between each pulse sequence), it is possible to bias it towards a particular component of the MR signal. Therefore, pulse sequences are described according to whether they emphasise differences in T_1, T_2 or proton density. For example, the imaging parameters used to acquire a T_1-weighted image ensure that tissue types with different T_1 times have the maximum contrast difference. White matter (which has a short T_1) appears relatively bright, while CSF (with a long T_1) appears dark on such a scan. In a T_2-weighted image, the scan sequence is designed to emphasise contrast between tissues with different T_2 times, such that, for example, CSF is very bright, compared to grey and white matter. In a proton density (PD)-weighted image, grey matter appears brighter than CSF, due to the greater density of protons in the former. Figure 3 shows T_1-weighted, T_2-weighted and PD-weighted images of a brain to demonstrate differences in tissue contrast seen with each type of scan.

Many texts and articles are available that provide more discussion of different pulse sequences for interested readers.

The MR signal can be localised to produce images of slices of the brain using a piece of equipment called a *gradient coil,* which produces a gradient in the magnetic field. By slightly changing the magnetic field, the Larmor frequency of protons differs slightly for each slice throughout the brain. It is therefore possible to apply the RF pulse at a frequency that will only excite protons in a single slice. Following the application of the RF pulse, two other gradients, a frequency encoding and a phase encoding gradient, are applied in order to localise the signal from each voxel in 3D space.

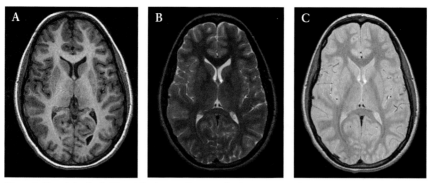

Figure 3. T$_1$-weighted (A), T$_2$-weighted (B) and PD-weighted (C) images of approximately the same slice of a brain.

With current MRI technology it is possible to acquire T$_1$-weighted 1.5 mm thick slices of the entire brain in around 6–10 minutes. Slice thickness is an important factor in the quality of MRI scans, because of the problem of partial volume effects. Partial volume effects occur when a voxel contains more than one tissue type: for example, at the boundary of grey and white matter, or between grey matter and CSF. This results in a blurring of the boundary between tissue. Thinner slices reduce this problem, as fewer voxels will contain a mixture of tissue types.

By comparison to CT, the superior resolution of MRI allows grey and white matter to be clearly distinguished and permits the visualization and assessment of midline and temporal lobe structures, such as the corpus callosum, hippocampus and amygdala, and subcortical structures, such as the caudate and thalamus, which are of interest in many psychiatric illnesses (Table 4).

MRI image planes
MRI allows flexibility in the choice of plane of image acquisition, and images are normally acquired in either the coronal (vertical), sagittal (side) or axial (horizontal) plane, although it is possible to acquire an image in any oblique plane. Figures 5–7 present MRI images in the standard radiologic manner, such that, on coronal and axial views, left is right and right is left. As can be seen, on coronal slices one can clearly visualize the ventricles, and temporal lobe structures (Figure 5); sagittal slices

Table 4. Advantages and limitations of MRI.

Advantages	Limitations
Good overall resolution, allowing visualization of midline structures which are not clearly visible with other techniques	The enclosed nature of the scanner and scanner noise may induce claustrophobic feelings
No known risk from magnetic fields	Increased scanning duration compared with CT increases the risk of problems such as movement artefacts which degrade scan quality
Provides excellent visibility of subcortical grey matter structures important in psychiatric illness, e.g. caudate and thalamus	Increased cost compared with CT

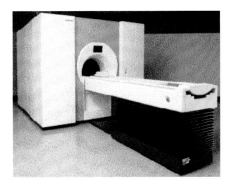

Figure 4. A typical MRI system. The chamber of the scanner resembles an open-ended tunnel. A magnetic field strength of 1.5 T is commonly used in clinical settings.

facilitate close examination of the brain stem, cerebellum and corpus callosum (Figure 6); and the axial view very clearly shows the cerebral hemispheres, ventricles and subcortical structures (Figure 7).

Recent advances in structural MRI

As can be seen from Figures 5–7, on MRI scans white matter appears relatively homogeneous. White matter consists primarily of myelinated bundles of axonal fibers connecting brain regions, and therefore is of interest in both neurological and psychiatric disorders. Recently, techniques have been developed that utilise MR technology to study the structure of these connecting bundles.

Diffusion-weighted imaging (DWI) is a technique that is sensitive to the movement of protons, and allows for the visualization of major white matter tracts connecting brain regions. DWI is based on the principle that, within fiber bundles, the movement of water molecules is restricted by myelin sheaths and cell membranes. This means that movement along the axonal bundles is easier than movement across them — referred to as diffusion anisotropy [1]. Diseases that interfere with these connecting bundles may be indicated by reduced anisotropy, which is thought to reflect reduced axonal integrity or density of fibers.

Pulse sequences have been developed that are sensitive to the movement of water molecules, such that areas of slow or restricted movement of water molecules (such as within an axonal bundle) have a high T_2 signal. If diffusion-weighted images are acquired, sensitive to diffusion to several orthogonal directions, it is possible not only to calculate the degree of diffusion anisotropy, but also the principal direction of diffusion at each voxel in white matter bundles. By studying the principal direction of diffusion at neighbouring voxels, it is possible to identify the directionality of major fiber tracts, allowing us to study both normal and abnormal connectivity [2].

Magnetization transfer imaging (MTI) also enables us to study white matter changes in vivo. Protons can be described as *free*, for example as constituents of water, or *bound*, as constituents of brain tissue such as myelin. In MTI, two T_2-weighted images are acquired: a conventional scan with an RF pulse applied at the normal Larmor frequency, and another where an RF pulse is applied at a frequency slightly different from the resonant frequency of free protons in water. This *off-resonance* pulse magnetizes bound, but not free, protons. Following

RIGHT   LEFT

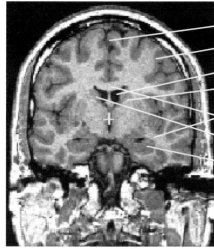

Interhemispheric fissure

Parietal lobe

Lateral ventricle

Internal capsule

Temporal lobe

Corpus callosum

Caudate nucleus

Hippocampus

Figure 5. T$_1$-weighted coronal view of a normal human brain, showing the image resolution possible with MRI. This scan shows the normal appearance of brain ventricles, sulcal spaces and temporal lobe regions.

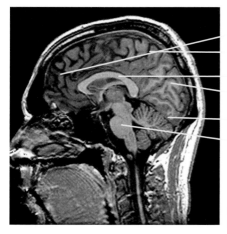

Frontal lobe

Parietal lobe

Corpus callosum

Occipital lobe

Cerebellum

Pons

Figure 6. The corpus callosum and cerebellum are clearly visible on the sagittal (left) view.

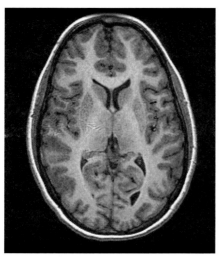

Figure 7. Axial view of the normal human brain.

cessation of this pulse, there is an exchange of magnetization from bound to free protons that leads to a decreased signal from free protons. By comparing the signal from the images with and without the off-resonance pulse it is possible to calculate the degree of magnetization transfer (MT). The degree of signal change between the images is determined by the number of bound protons, as more bound protons lead to greater MT and to a greater reduction in the signal from free protons. White matter changes in MT are believed to be principally sensitive to changes in myelination of axonal bundles, such that reduced MT is thought to reflect decreased myelination [3].

Although they are relatively new techniques, both DWI and MTI have already been applied successfully to the study of a number of neurological conditions such as multiple sclerosis, epilepsy and cerebral ischaemia [4]. As well as their clinical applications, DWI and MTI should aid our understanding of the complex connections between brain regions, and how these may be affected by illnesses such as schizophrenia.

References

1.   Lim KO, Hedehus M, Moseley M et al. Compromised white matter tract integrity inferred from diffusion tensor imaging. *Arch Gen Psychiatry* 1999;56:367–74.
2.   Jones DK, Horsfield MA, Simmons A. Optimal strategies for measuring diffusion in anisotropic systems by magnetic resonance imaging. *Magn Reson Med* 1999;42(3):515–25.
3.   Rademacher J, Engelbrecht V, Burgel U et al. Measuring in vivo myelination of human white matter fiber tracts with magnetization transfer MR. *Neuroimage* 1999;9(4):393–406.
4.   Rowley HA, Grant PE, Roberts TP. Diffusion MR imaging. Theory and applications. *Neuroimaging Clin N Am* 1999;9(2):343–61.

CHAPTER 2

Functional Brain Imaging

The ability to visualize brain structure has greatly advanced our knowledge of psychiatric disorders. However, this information is of relatively little use unless it can be integrated with knowledge of how the brain works. As will be discussed later, it is clear that brain function is abnormal in psychiatric disorders such as schizophrenia, and over the last two decades a number of techniques have been developed to enable us to study the workings of the brain in vivo.

Positron emission tomography

Positron emission tomography (PET) is a technique that has transformed our understanding of neural function and chemistry. PET facilitates the evaluation of cerebral metabolic activity and blood flow, and neurotransmitter receptor number and function (Table 1). PET has a number of clinical applications — for example, in diagnosing brain tumours and assessing the effects of cerebral infarction. However, given the need for an on-site cyclotron unit to produce the receptor ligand (radionuclide), it has very limited availability and is most commonly used for research.

Table 1. Applications of PET in psychiatry and contraindications for the technique.

Applications in psychiatry	Contraindications
Quantifying neurotransmitter receptors and visualizing the sites of action of drugs	Uses radioactive substances, thus the level of radiation exposure is an important determinant of use
Measurement of cerebral glucose metabolism and regional cerebral blood flow can be used to study resting brain activity, or to map cerebral activation during cognitive or motor tasks	Known allergic or anaphylactic reactions to radioligands, e.g. [^{11}C]raclopride, [^{11}C]N-methyl-spiperone, [^{18}F]deoxyglucose and ^{15}O-labelled water

Principles of PET

Positron emission is a very rapid form of radioactive decay. In PET, a radioactive substance is attached to either a normal body substance (e.g. glucose) or a drug (in the case of receptor binding). When labelled with the positron-emitting chemical, it becomes known as a radioactive tracer or radionuclide. The tracer is then injected into the bloodstream of the subject, where it crosses the blood-brain barrier and circulates within the cerebrovasculature. As it decays, the tracer emits positrons, which interact with surrounding electrons in a so-called *annihilation reaction* to produce two gamma-ray photons oriented at 180° to each other [1]. The PET scanner has an array of receptors surrounding the head that detect these emissions (Figure 1). It is only the simultaneous arrival of two photons at opposite detectors that is recorded as a signal, and this permits the localization of emissions, since the reaction must have occurred on a line between the two detectors. Computer reconstruction provides a tomographic image of the distribution of the tracer.

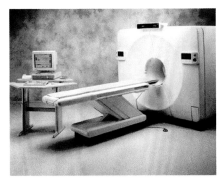

Figure 1. A typical clinical PET imaging suite.

PET imaging of receptor function

The ability to understand in vivo brain chemistry, and to investigate the effects of different drugs on brain chemistry, has revolutionized psychopharmacology. The development of PET and single photon emission computed tomography (SPECT) has allowed researchers to investigate neurotransmitter receptors and transporters directly. Both technologies involve injecting a subject with a radiolabelled substance that has a high affinity and specificity for the receptor under study. As the tracer travels around the brain, it binds to receptors. The emissions from the radiolabelled ligand over time can be measured and localized to give an indication of where the substance is binding, and how strongly. This reflects receptor distribution and allows quantification. This technique can also be used to study the site of action of drugs. For example, if a subject is given a drug that selectively blocks dopamine D_2 receptors, and is then given a PET scan with [^{11}C]raclopride (a D_2 receptor ligand), the subject will show reduced binding of the ligand, as some of the D_2 receptors have already been occupied by the drug. Kegeles and Mann provide an excellent review of PET and SPECT imaging [2].

Advances in PET imaging of receptor function

Some authors have hypothesized that the neurochemical disturbance in illnesses such as schizophrenia may not simply be a dysfunction in one transmitter system but may instead reflect abnormal modulation of one system by another [3]. The ability to visualize modulation of one neurotransmitter system by another is a huge step forward in elucidating the chemical disturbances involved in psychiatric disorders. As an example of this, Smith and co-workers investigated the effects of ketamine — a known psychogenic drug that binds to the glutamate N-methyl-D-aspartate (NMDA) receptor — on dopamine binding [4]. They found that administration of ketamine led to reduced binding of [^{11}C]raclopride in the striatum, showing that glutamate receptors could significantly affect dopamine function. In terms of understanding neurotransmitter interactions and possible abnormalities in psychiatric disorders, this is an exciting development.

PET imaging of regional cerebral blood flow

Mapping human brain function is one of the recent exciting applications of PET technology. With a spatial resolution of 3–5 mm, PET can provide a detailed picture of the functional neuroanatomy of motor function or cognitive processes such as language, memory, attention and emotion (Table 2). Increased neuronal activity in an area of the brain is paralleled by an increase in blood supply. Images of regional cerebral blood flow (rCBF) are obtained by using water labelled with an oxygen isotope: [^{15}O]H$_2$O. When a particular region is activated, it needs more blood; therefore, by tracking the emissions from the radiolabelled water it is possible to track which regions are activated during specific cognitive or motor tasks.

Figure 2 shows a reconstructed PET image of rCBF during a finger-tracking task. From this type of image it is possible to calculate regions of increased activation between subject groups or experimental conditions (Figure 3).

PET imaging of glucose metabolism

Glucose is the principal source of energy for neurones. Abnormal glucose metabolism is an indication of underlying pathology and can be detected by PET imaging using an [^{18}F]deoxyglucose tracer. Regional glucose metabolism can be assessed with PET during the resting state, or during performance of a cognitive task, by monitoring emissions from the tracer as it is metabolized. Thus, as with studies of rCBF it is possible to identify regions activated by particular tasks.

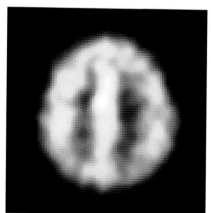

Figure 2. PET image of rCBF during a finger-tracking task.
Image courtesy of Dr Ivo Dinov & Dr Michael Mega, Laboratory of Neuroimaging (LONI), UCLA, USA.

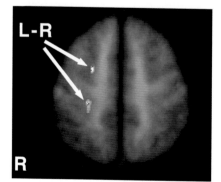
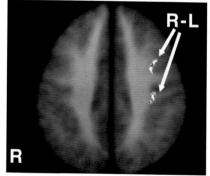

Figure 3. (From left to right) Regions of increased cerebral activation during left-hand and right-hand finger tracking. Images are in radiographic orientation.
Image courtesy of Dr Ivo Dinov & Dr Michael Mega, Laboratory of Neuroimaging (LONI), UCLA, USA.

Table 2. Advantages and limitations of PET imaging.

Advantages	Limitations
Facilitates the assessment of receptor distribution in the brain	A local radiochemistry department is required for production of radiotracer substances, since the half-life of these compounds is short. PET is therefore expensive and unlikely to be available for routine clinical use
Measurement of cerebral blood flow during neuropsychological testing allows mapping of regions of cerebral activation during cognitive or motor tasks	
PET cerebral glucose metabolism can reflect resting brain activity, or metabolism during a cognitive task	Radiation dose limits repeated scanning. Using low doses of radiotracer minimizes this problem, but prolongs scanning time
Improved anatomic localization of activity is possible by overlaying PET scan information on to MRI images	Low spatial and temporal resolution when compared with functional MRI

Single photon emission computed tomography

SPECT is a similar technique to PET, and may be used for direct measurement of central neurochemical systems in vivo. It is based on single photon emissions from decaying radionuclides. Like PET, SPECT allows us to study neurotransmitter receptors, the site of action of psychotropic drugs and the functional effects of psychiatric illness on regional brain activity (Table 3). SPECT ligands generally have a longer half-life than those used in PET, and so there is no need for an on-site cyclotron unit. Therefore, compared with PET, SPECT is a cheaper and more widely available technique. However, it is hampered by lower spatial resolution (Table 4).

Principles of SPECT

In SPECT, the decay of a radionuclide results in the emission of a single gamma-ray photon. Like CT (see Chapter 1), in SPECT a detector rotates around the subject, stopping at regular intervals to record the gamma emissions. Modern SPECT scanners may consist of two or three gamma cameras to detect emissions. The gamma camera comprises a collimator, detectors and a crystal. The collimator consists of thousands of channels through which the gamma rays can pass, and its function is to ensure that only emissions that are perpendicular to the angle of the camera are detected. This permits the localization of the emissions. (In PET this is

Table 3. Applications of SPECT in psychiatry and contraindications for the technique.

Applications in psychiatry	Contraindications
Localization of brain receptor populations	Uses radioactive substances, thus the level of radiation exposure is an important determinant of use
Determination of brain receptor occupancy by psychotropic drugs	
Investigation of effects of drugs on brain receptors	Known allergic or anaphylactic reactions to radioligands, e.g. [^{11}C]raclopride, [^{11}C]N-methyl-spiperone, [^{18}F]deoxyglucose and ^{15}O-labelled water
Visualization of brain activity during task performance	

achieved naturally, as the two gamma rays travel on a straight line away from each other, meaning that their origin can be traced back along that line.) The gamma rays interact with the crystal, producing a signal, which is recorded by a grid of detectors behind the crystal. The distribution of the radiotracer can then be displayed for localization and quantification of receptor binding (Figures 4 and 5) or for localization of functional activation.

Table 4. Advantages and limitations of SPECT.

Advantages	Limitations
Less expensive then PET imaging because of the longer half-life of tracers. Unlike in PET, an on-site cyclotron unit is not needed, therefore it is a more widely available technique	Involves the use of intravenous radiolabelled substances
An expanding range of radiotracer compounds with long half-life values enhances the range of SPECT applications	The spatial resolution of SPECT (8–10 mm) is not as good as that of PET — precise localization is not possible
State-of-the-art cameras and collimators offer improved spatial resolution	

SPECT imaging of receptor activity
PET and SPECT have been instrumental in giving scientists and clinicians a greater understanding of the site of drug action. They help us to understand the degree of receptor occupancy, the time required for drug uptake at receptors and the clinical consequences thereof. This provides information on the drug dose required to produce the degree of receptor occupancy necessary for clinical efficacy — and the level that induces side-effects — thus impacting directly on patient care and management.

SPECT imaging of brain function
As with PET, SPECT allows for the visualization of regional brain activity during performance of a task. As mentioned above, the spatial resolution of SPECT is

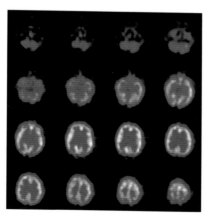

Figure 4. SPECT image of the distribution of [^{123}I]iomazenil, which labels GABA-benzodiazepine receptors (brighter colour indicates stronger binding). The occipital area displays the highest level of [^{123}I]iomazenil uptake, indicating a high level of receptor distribution.
Image courtesy of Dr Anne Lingford-Hughes, Department of Psychological Medicine, Institute of Psychiatry, London, UK.

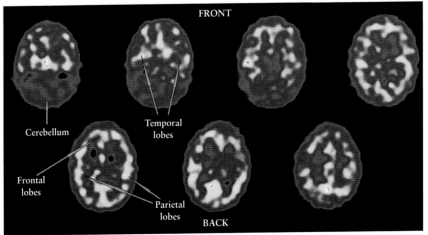

Figure 5. SPECT scan of a normal control, demonstrating binding of the [^{123}I]-5-I-R91150 ligand to 5-HT$_{2A}$ receptors. As can be seen, there is virtually no binding in the cerebellum, indicating a lack of receptors, but a high level of binding in all cortical regions.
Reproduced with permission from Travis MJ, Busatto GF, Pilowsky LS et al. 5-HT$_{2A}$ receptor blockade in schizophrenic patients treated with risperidone or clozapine. A single photon emission tomography (SPET) using the novel 5-HT$_{2A}$ ligand [^{123}I]-5-I-R-91150. Br J Psychiat 1998;173:236–42.

poorer than that of PET (8–10 mm, as compared with 4–5 mm); however, it is cheaper, and more widely available. As with PET imaging of blood flow, the radiolabelled substance, usually 99mTechnetium-hexamethylpropylene amine oxime (Tc-HMPAO-99m), is injected into the bloodstream and, as it decays, the gamma emissions are monitored by the SPECT camera. This allows for the localization of brain activity during cognitive or motor tasks.

Functional magnetic resonance imaging

Probably the greatest advance in psychiatric neuroimaging of the last few years has been the development of functional MRI (fMRI). With spatial resolution as good as 1 mm, and temporal resolution of one second or less, it is far superior to PET. Functional MRI affords the possibility of mapping cognitive function to very precise neuroanatomic structures, helping to identify structures and functional networks that may be abnormal in psychiatric illnesses. While PET requires the injection of radiolabelled substances, fMRI is entirely non-invasive. This allows for repeated scanning and longitudinal studies, which are very restricted with PET.

Applications of fMRI

Functional MRI allows for very precise mapping of cognitive functions onto brain structure. Although fMRI is currently primarily used as a research tool to aid our understanding of psychiatric disorders, in the future it is likely to become more widely used in clinical care. An excellent introduction to clinical applications of fMRI is given by Haughton et al [5]. The current primary clinical application of fMRI is in localizing brain function in patients with tumours who are candidates for neurosurgery or to alleviate symptoms of epilepsy. In the case of tumour removal, for example, it is important to ensure that surgery will not result in a post-operative deficit — fMRI allows us to map cognitive and motor functions in order to identify what regions must be avoided and what functions may be at risk from surgery. Prior to surgery for epilepsy, patients are usually tested to identify which hemisphere is dominant for language, in order to ensure functional preservation. Traditionally, this has been done by anaesthetizing each hemisphere in turn (usually with an injection of sodium amytal), and then conducting neuropsychological tests. Functional MRI offers the potential of localizing brain function in these patients in a non-invasive and more accurate way.

Contraindications for fMRI

Functional MRI can be undertaken in any appropriately equipped MRI scanner; contraindications, therefore, are the same as for MRI.

Principles of fMRI

Like structural MRI, fMRI utilizes the magnetic properties of protons. It relies on the observation that it is possible to differentiate the MR signal from activated and non-activated regions of the brain. Although some fMRI studies use exogenous substances such as gadolinium in order to produce a clear signal change in activated regions, most prefer to use a non-invasive approach that capitalizes on the endogenous changes in the brain produced by functional activation. In this case, the fMRI signal is based on the natural haemodynamic response to increased activity in a particular brain region. At its simplest, it works by detecting changes in blood oxygenation. Good introductions to fMRI are available [6-8].

As explained in Chapter 1, when placed in a strong magnetic field, the magnetic moments of hydrogen nuclei line up parallel to the field. When a radio-frequency (RF) pulse is applied, this alignment is disturbed. After removal of the pulse, the moments reorient parallel to the field. The time for the spins to dephase is called T_2 (transverse relaxation), and is affected by the surrounding tissue type, and, most importantly, by local variation in magnetic field strength. The T_2 relaxation time is affected by the surrounding tissue type and, most importantly, by local variation in magnetic field strength. Local field inhomogeneity leads to reduced T_2 time, called T_2^*. The variation in T_2^* relaxation time induced by local variations in magnetic field strength is the key to fMRI.

When the neurones in a particular brain region are activated, this is accompanied by increased blood flow to the active region. Thus, there is an increase in oxygenated blood (blood containing oxyhaemoglobin) to satisfy the requirements of the activated region. However, this supply of oxygenated blood outstrips the metabolic usage of the oxygen, resulting in a temporary over-supply. Oxygenated blood and deoxygenated blood have very different magnetic properties, in that deoxygenated blood is paramagnetic (i.e. although nonmagnetic, it behaves magnetically in the presence of an external field such as an MRI scanner), and so increases local magnetic field inhomogeneity. Activity in a cerebral region alters the local magnetic field by increasing the ratio of oxygenated to deoxygenated blood, thereby decreasing the paramagnetic effects of deoxyhaemoglobin. This leads to a longer T_2^* relaxation time, producing a stronger signal from the active region, compared to its non-active state [9]. Because the signal is dependent on changes in blood oxygenation levels, this method has been termed the 'blood-oxygenation-level-dependent' or 'BOLD' effect. The principles of fMRI are illustrated in Figure 6.

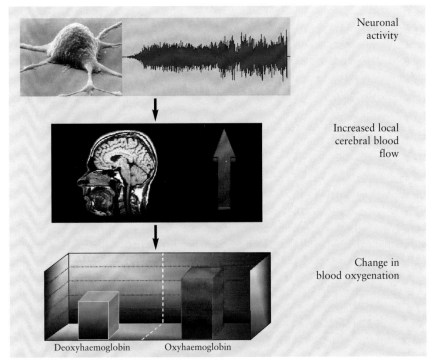

Neuronal
activity

Increased local
cerebral blood
flow

Change in
blood oxygenation

Deoxyhaemoglobin   Oxyhaemoglobin

Figure 6. The principles of fMRI.
Image courtesy of Garry Honey, Section of Cognitive Psychopharmacology, Institute of Psychiatry, London, UK.

Mapping functional activation on to brain structure

In order to localize regions of activation accurately, scans are usually transformed into so-called 'stereotactic space', usually corresponding to the atlas of Talairach and Tournoux [10]. This is a standard space that minimizes variability between scans by warping them into structural correspondence with a template image. This removes the effects of normal variation in brain anatomy, ensuring that structures from many subjects are located at the same point. Activation can be averaged across a group of subjects to produce a group map of brain activity (Figure 7). It is then possible to compare patterns of brain activation between subject groups, or between experimental conditions.

Future developments in fMRI

Most current fMRI experiments are of the so-called block or box-car design. This involves alternating experimental paradigms consisting of a series of trials with a resting state, in order to visualize regional activation, or it can involve alternating different experimental tasks in order to tease out the subcomponents of a functional network. Images are constantly acquired during each block. One development that will greatly extend the utility of fMRI is event-related fMRI. This involves measuring the signal change (activation) resulting from a single trial or stimulus presentation, and allows for much more sensitive experimental paradigms than are possible with blocked designs. This sort of experimental design is not possible with PET or SPECT, due to the relatively prolonged activity that is needed in order to detect change with these methods. Event-related fMRI will allow researchers to

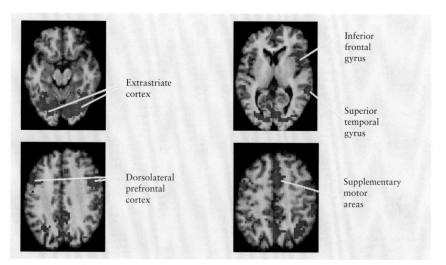

Figure 7. Brain activity in a group of healthy subjects during a language task, superimposed onto a template image. *Image courtesy of Garry Honey, Section of Cognitive Psychopharmacology, Institute of Psychiatry, London, UK.*

study the temporal nature of changes in brain activity with a resolution in the order of milliseconds, as changes in blood oxygenation are detectable very quickly following presentation of a stimulus. This level of temporal resolution has only previously been available with electrophysiological recording techniques, which lack the spatial resolution of fMRI. Examining the haemodynamic response to single events allows us, for example, to identify regions involved in planning and then execute a motor response. Excellent introductions to event-related fMRI are available [11,12].

Generally, data are acquired in an fMRI scan and analysed later. Recent technical advances allow for real-time analysis, such that information on a subject's brain activity is available almost instantaneously. This should greatly increase the clinical applicability of fMRI by rapidly providing information that would be useful for surgical planning, or disease and treatment monitoring [8].

Most structural and functional MRI studies are currently carried out on 1.5 Tesla scanners. This is adequate for most tasks. However, higher-field-strength scanners, e.g. 3.0 or 4.0 T, allow for finer anatomic resolution, indicating regions of activation more precisely. At 1.5 T, the signal increase seen with increased activation is only of the order of 2–5%; however, the signal is amplified by about 15% with a 4.0 T magnet [6].

Magnetic resonance spectroscopy

Magnetic resonance spectroscopy (MRS) is a non-invasive imaging technique that is used to study in vivo neurochemistry. While PET and SPECT provide information on neurotransmitter receptors, and fMRI allows us to investigate the functional organization of the brain, MRS is used to study the metabolites of a range of substances involved in basic biochemical processes. MRS has applications in the study of basic brain processes, disease diagnosis and treatment monitoring, and can identify neurochemical abnormalities in the absence of structural changes (Table 5).

Table 5. Applications of MRS in psychiatry and contraindications for the technique.

Applications in psychiatry	Contraindications
Study of amino acids, neurotransmitters and their metabolites, and compounds involved in brain energy processes	Biomedical implants with ferromagnetic properties including defibrillators, neural stimulators, infusion pumps, cochlear implants, aneurysm clips, metallic aortic stents, plates and prostheses
Assessment of neuronal membrane metabolism	
May be used in conjunction with MRI, thus offering simultaneous study of brain structure and function	Pacemakers or a history of invasive heart surgery
A potential aid in early diagnosis and subsequent monitoring of illness	Pregnancy, particularly during the first trimester
Determination of pharmacokinetic and pharmacodynamic properties of psychiatric drugs	Previous operations to the head, neck or spinal area

Principles of MRS

MRS permits the in vivo assessment of levels of molecules involved in a variety of neural processes, including neurotransmitters, components of cell membranes and compounds related to energy usage. However, MRS only allows detection in approximately the millimolar range; therefore, many interesting metabolites remain undetectable by MRS because of the low levels at which they are present (Table 6).

Table 6. Advantages and limitations of MRS imaging.

Advantages of MRS	Limitations of MRS
Offers a relatively sophisticated means of assessing brain metabolism	Suffers from a relative lack of sensitivity — the low millimolar concentrations of some metabolites are not detectable
Potential aid in early diagnosis and subsequent monitoring of illness	Transient biochemical changes are difficult to detect
Allows determination of pharmacokinetic and pharmacodynamic properties of psychiatric drugs	Poor resolution properties make it difficult to distinguish between biochemically similar compounds
	Prone to partial volume effects

During the MRS scanning procedure, a conventional structural scan is usually acquired. This is then used in order to identify a region-of-interest from which MRS signals will be measured. As with MRI, the spins of hydrogen nuclei line up in the scanner, parallel to the direction of the magnet. RF pulses are applied and cause a change in the orientation of the spins. When the RF pulses are removed, the spins of the nuclei return to their original alignment (relaxation).

The signal emitted during relaxation yields a spectrum displaying the intensity of different chemical entities and the shift in resonant frequency — in parts per million (ppm) — relative to a standard substance. Although the peaks visible on an MRS spectrum are all signals from the same type of atom, e.g. hydrogen atoms for ¹H spectroscopy, the resonant frequency of the nuclei as they relax to their original orientation is strongly influenced by variations in local magnetic fields, so that the resonant frequency for the same atom will be different according to the molecule (chemical environment) it is part of. This produces the different peaks on an MRS spectrum, and is known as *chemical shift* [13].

Although MRS is a widely used clinical and research tool, it has a number of limitations. Firstly, it is relatively insensitive; thus it is not possible to study some potentially interesting metabolites due to their low concentrations in tissue. Secondly, it is difficult to assign the effects of different chemicals to their corresponding peaks on an MRS spectrum, although recent advances have begun to overcome this problem (see below).

Types of MRS
Initial studies in the mid-1980s were performed using proton (¹H) MRS. Due to technological advances, it is now possible to do in vivo MRS with phosphorus (³¹P), carbon-13 (¹³C), fluorine (¹⁹F) and lithium (⁷Li).

Proton magnetic resonance spectroscopy (¹H MRS)
Due to the abundance of hydrogen-containing molecules in the body, proton spectroscopy should theoretically be a relatively easy technique. In reality, the abundance of hydrogen molecules from water in the brain can drown out the signal from interesting compounds. This problem can be overcome by using sequences that suppress the water signal.

Proton spectroscopy allows for the detection of a large array of hydrogen-containing compounds. The results of proton spectroscopy are presented as a series of peaks (Figure 8):

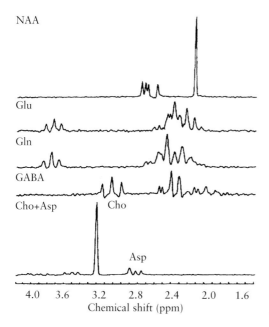

Figure 8. MRS spectrum showing the position of metabolites detected by ¹H (proton) spectroscopy, as determined by their chemical shift pattern.

Brain Imaging in Schizophrenia

- N-acetyl aspartate (NAA) — proposed to be a marker of neuronal and axonal integrity; a reduced NAA signal indicates reduced neuronal density, or neuronal or axonal dysfunction [14]
- Creatine (Cr) and phosphocreatine (PCr) — chemicals linked to energy states; altered levels may indicate reduced regional activity
- Choline (Cho) — the choline constituents are believed to be related to membrane activity; abnormalities may indicate some kind of cellular pathology
- Glutamine (Gln), glutamate, alanine, aspartate (Asp) and gamma aminobutyric acid (GABA) — alterations in the levels of these substances and their metabolites may indicate neurotransmitter dysfunction
- Glucose (Glu) and lactate — alterations in the levels of these chemicals may indicate regional metabolic dysfunction

Phosphorus spectroscopy (^{31}P MRS)

Phosphorus spectroscopy facilitates direct measurement of brain phospholipids and high-energy phosphate metabolism (Figure 9):

- Phosphomonoesters (PME) and phosphodiesters (PDE) — metabolites of the precursors and breakdown products of cell membrane constituents
- Phosphocreatine (PCr), nucleoside triphosphates (e.g. adenosine triphosphate [ATP]) and inorganic phosphates (Pi) — all indicators of energy metabolism; levels of these metabolites provide an overall measure of neuronal well-being and activity

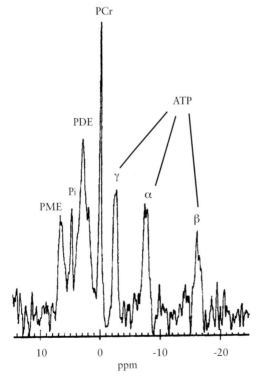

Figure 9. ^{31}P (phosphorus) MRS spectrum from the frontal lobe of a normal human brain. The phosphomonoester (PME), phosphodiester (PDE), high-energy phosphate (ATP) and phosphocreatine (PCr) metabolite peaks are shown.

Future developments in MRS

As with both structural and functional MRI, MRS is increasingly being used in routine clinical practice to aid diagnosis and treatment of a variety of neurological conditions. A detailed review of the clinical uses of MRS is given by Rudkin and Arnold [15]. To date, the primary clinical use of MRS has been in the diagnosis of brain tumours. Although conventional imaging techniques such as CT and MRI can be used to detect a tumour, they cannot distinguish between tumour types. A number of studies have now shown that different types and grades of tumour have a different spectroscopic pattern [16], and so can be diagnosed in a non-invasive way. MRS may also be useful in the clinical management of multiple sclerosis, which is characterized by the demyelination of axons. White matter lesions are not always identifiable using conventional MRI; however, it has been shown that MRS can identify lesions even before they become visible on MRI scans. With both these disorders, research is currently investigating whether MRS may be used as a way of monitoring and predicting treatment response. Evidence of the potential of MRS for monitoring treatment effects has come from studies of amyotrophic lateral sclerosis (ALS). In ALS, neurones in the motor cortex die, and it has been demonstrated that patients with ALS show reduced levels of NAA. Interestingly, a recent study showed that patients treated with a glutamate antagonist have increased levels of NAA, indicating that some neuronal damage may be reversible, and that this can be detected with MRS [17]. As MR imaging becomes more widely available in hospitals, these sorts of techniques are likely to have a major impact on the clinical care of patients with neurological disorders.

Traditionally, MRS has been limited by the fact that many metabolites are indistinguishable from each other on an MRS spectrum. For example, the PME and PDE peaks seen in ^{31}P spectroscopy are formed from the signal from a variety of metabolites containing these chemical groups. One technique that can remove this problem is proton-decoupled spectroscopy [18], which has been shown to separate out the contribution of different components to the PME and PDE peaks.

Using MRS, it is possible to measure exogenous compounds such as ^{19}F and ^{13}C. Many of the drugs used in clinical psychiatry are fluorinated compounds, and therefore it should be possible to measure in vivo levels of antipsychotic and antidepressant medications [19]. Determining the pharmacokinetics of psychoactive drugs is important in assessing and/or predicting treatment response. As clinical responses generally have a slower onset, by allowing us to identify local drug concentrations, MRS offers the possibility of immediately assessing the effects of drug treatment on brain activity.

References

1. Bench CA, Spence SA, Bench CJ, Spence SA. PET blood flow studies in schizophrenia. *J Adv Schizophr Brain Res* 1998;**1**(3):71–7. *J Adv Schizophr Brain Res* 1998;**1**(3):71–7.
2. Kegeles LS, Mann JJ. In vivo imaging of neurotransmitter systems using radiolabelled receptor ligands. *Neuropsychopharmacology* 1997;**17**:293–307.
3. Remington G, Kapur S. D$_2$ and 5-HT$_2$ receptor effects of antipsychotics: bridging basic and clinical findings using PET. *J Clin Psychiatry* 1999;**60**(Suppl 10):15–9.
4. Smith GS, Schloesser R, Brodie JD et al. Glutamate modulation of dopamine measured in vivo with positron emission tomography (PET) and ^{11}C-raclopride in normal human subjects. *Neuropsychopharmacology* 1998;**18**:18–25.

5.   Haughton VM, Turski PA Meyerand B et al. The clinical applications of functional MR imaging. *Neuroimaging Clin N Am* 1999;**9**(2):285–93.
6.   Cohen MS, Bookheimer SY. Localization of brain function using magnetic resonance imaging. *Trends Neurosci* 1994;**17**:268–77.
7.   Kindermann SS, Karimi A, Symonds L et al. Review of functional magnetic resonance imaging in schizophrenia. *Schizophr Res* 1997;**27**:143–56.
8.   Longworth CE, Honey G, Sharma T. Science, medicine and the future: functional magnetic resonance imaging in neuropsychiatry. *Br Med J* 1999;**319**:1551–4.
9.   Honey G, Sharma T. Functional magnetic resonance imaging: a window on the brain and the future of schizophrenia research. *J Adv Schizophr Brain Res* 1999;**1**(4):106–110.
10. Talairach J, Tournoux P. A Co-planar Stereotaxic Map of the Human Brain. Germany: Thieme 1988.
11. Rosen BR, Buckner RL, Dale AM. Event-related functional MRI: past, present and future. *Proc Natl Acad Sci USA* 1998;**95**(3):773–80.
12. Menon RS, Kim SG. Spatial and temporal limits in cognitive neuroimaging with fMRI. *Trends Cogn Sci* 1999;**3**:207–16.
13. Frangou S, Williams SC. Magnetic resonance spectroscopy in psychiatry: basic principles and applications. *Br Med Bull* 1996;**52**:474–85.
14. Kegeles LS, Humaran TJ, Mann JJ. In vivo neurochemistry of the brain in schizophrenia as revealed by magnetic resonance spectroscopy. *Biol Psychiatry* 1998;**44**:382–98.
15. Rudkin TM, Arnold DL. Proton magnetic resonance spectroscopy for the diagnosis and management of cerebral disorders. *Arch Neurol* 1999;**56**(8):919–26.
16. Preul MC, Caramanos Z, Collins DL et al. Accurate, noninvasive diagnosis of human brain tumors by using proton magnetic resonance spectroscopy. *Nature Med* 1996;**2**(3):323–5.
17. Kalra S, Cashman NR, Genge A et al. Recovery of N-acetylaspartate in corticomotor neurons of patients with ALS after riluzole therapy. *Neuroreport* 1998;**9**(8):1757–61.
18. Potwarka JJ, Drost DJ, Williamson PC et al. A ^{1}H-decoupled ^{31}P chemical shift imaging study of medicated schizophrenic patients and healthy controls. *Biol Psychiatry* 1999;**45**:687–93.
19. Kato T, Inubushi T, Kato N. Magnetic resonance spectroscopy in affective disorders. *J Neuropsychiatry Clin Neurosci* 1998;**10**(2):133–47.

CHAPTER 3
Structural Brain Imaging in Schizophrenia

Computed tomographic imaging in schizophrenia

The first CT study of schizophrenia by Johnstone et al. was a landmark paper that changed our understanding of the disorder by demonstrating that it had an identifiable biological basis [1]. Although computed tomography (CT) has generally been superseded by magnetic resonance imaging (MRI) as a research tool, it is still used owing to its lower cost, wider availability and reduced scanning time.

The predominant finding of CT studies in schizophrenia is enlargement of the ventricles and cortical sulci, such as the sylvian fissure [2] together with widespread cortical [3] and cerebellar atrophy [4]. Other studies have shown that schizophrenics with significant sulcal enlargement have impaired cognitive functioning [5], while ventricular enlargement has been found to be associated with longer illness duration and more severe negative symptoms, as well as with impaired cognitive functioning [6]. These structural changes have also been linked with a history of obstetric complications [7] and maternal influenza during pregnancy [8]. A recent longitudinal study using CT scans taken 4 years apart identified two separate subgroups of schizophrenics [9]. One group, termed 'Kraepelinian', defined on the basis of very low social functioning and self-care, showed a marked increase in ventricular volume over the 4 years. In contrast, the second group, termed 'non-Kraepelinian', showed no significant change in ventricular volume between the two scans.

Magnetic resonance imaging in schizophrenia

Features of MRI in schizophrenia

The increased sensitivity and resolution afforded by MRI have revolutionized the types of research that can be carried out into brain structure in schizophrenia. It is now possible to study patients during their first psychotic episode, or after years of chronic illness, to examine macroscopic progressive change, or the effects of different types of antipsychotic medication. These advances have significantly enhanced our understanding of schizophrenia.

As with CT, the most consistent finding of MRI research into schizophrenia is of lateral and third ventricle enlargement (Figure 1) [10]. This is present in first-episode patients [11,12], indicating that it may be a pre-existing abnormality, and it may be a genetic marker for the illness (see Chapter 5) [13]. Many structures and regions are smaller in the brains of schizophrenics. Reduced cerebral volume has been reported — although contradictory reports exist [14,15] — and reduced cortical grey matter volume is also a common finding [16,17]. For a review and a meta-analysis of the literature on structural brain changes in schizophrenia, see McCarley et al.[15] and Wright et al. [18]

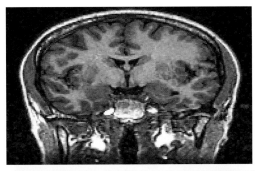

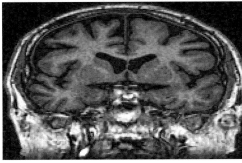

Figure 1. MRI scan of the brain of a normal control (top) and a schizophrenic (bottom). The schizophrenic brain shows marked ventricular and sulcal enlargement.

Frontal lobes and schizophrenia

Phylogenetically, the frontal lobes are the most recently developed regions of the brain. They demonstrate remarkable functional heterogeneity and are involved in higher order cognitive functions such as language, learning, memory and emotion. As will be discussed in Chapter 4, functional imaging techniques have indicated that schizophrenia may be characterized by frontal lobe abnormalities. Although the literature from structural imaging studies is controversial[15], there is some evidence of reduced frontal lobe volume[11]. However, given the functional heterogeneity of the frontal lobes, research is increasingly trying to subdivide them into functionally relevant subregions, as this may be more informative about abnormalities in schizophrenia.

A recent study reported that schizophrenics showed reduced total prefrontal volume, together with reduced volume of the left and right inferior prefrontal cortex[19]. Another study reported reduced grey matter in the left dorsolateral prefrontal cortex, a region heavily involved in executive cognitive functions (Figure 2)[20]. There is also evidence of grey matter loss in other frontal regions, including the middle frontal gyrus, and the medial-frontal and orbitofrontal cortices[21]. However, two other studies that examined subdivisions of the prefrontal cortex found no significant differences between schizophrenics and controls[22,23].

Interestingly, some recent research has suggested that structural abnormalities in the frontal lobes may be more complex than reductions in grey matter. Two studies have shown that some frontal lobe regions may actually be enlarged in the brains of schizophrenics[21,24]. During prenatal brain development, more neurones are produced than are needed. Neurones migrate to cortical regions, and attempt to form connections with other regions. Neurones that do not make appropriate connections are pruned through a process of programmed cell death. It has been suggested that this is due to abnormal cortical pruning during development, possibly caused by inappropriate development of reciprocally connected regions. As the study of frontal lobes is still in its infancy, very little is known about how prefrontal abnormalities may be linked to symptom profile and cognitive functioning.

Temporal lobe structures and schizophrenia

Temporal lobe structures have been a particular focus of research into structural abnormalities in schizophrenia, as some authors have argued that the underlying pathology of the illness is linked to this region [25]. The evidence for temporal lobe changes is much more extensive and consistent than for frontal lobe abnormalities. Many studies have reported reduced temporal lobe volume in schizophrenia [26], with some evidence that this is primarily a left-sided effect [27]. Two

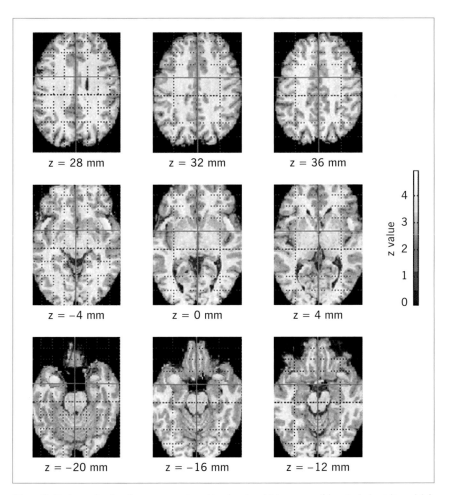

Figure 2. Regions of reduced grey matter in schizophrenics. Major areas of loss include right and left temporal poles and insula, right amygdala and left dorsolateral prefrontal cortex.
Reproduced with permission from Wright IC, Ellison ZR, Sharma T et al. Mapping of grey matter changes in schizophrenia. Schizophr Res 1999;35:1–14.

recent studies [20,21] have reported grey matter reductions in the insula (see Figure 2), which like many temporal lobe structures is strongly connected with prefrontal regions.

The limbic system is a network of structures that are involved in learning, memory and emotion, and is often implicated in schizophrenic pathology. As part of the limbic system, the hippocampus and amygdala have been extensively studied in schizophrenia (see Nelson et al.[28] for review and meta-analysis). Reduced volume of the hippocampus and parahippocampal gyrus has been regularly reported [15,28], although there are contradictory findings [29]. Again, some studies have indicated that this is a predominantly left-sided phenomenon [30], while others have reported bilateral volume reductions [31]. Reduced amygdala volume is a less consistent finding. Although some researchers have reported amygdala abnormalities [20], many studies measure the hippocampus and amygdala together, as the hippocampus-amygdala complex [32], and this may obscure potential differences.

The superior temporal gyrus (STG) is believed to be involved in language function and is therefore of particular interest in schizophrenia. Data are currently equivocal: some studies have reported reduced STG volume in schizophrenics [33] — particularly on the left side [34] — but there have been contradictory findings [35]. Studies that examined STG grey matter only have much more consistently reported tissue loss [15,36].

Substantial effort has been devoted to identifying functional consequences of these structural changes. Consistent relationships have been found between the volume of temporal lobe structures and positive symptoms of schizophrenia. In particular, reduced volume of the STG has also been associated with severity of positive symptoms such as thought disorder and hallucinations [37–39]. Given that the STG contains the primary auditory cortex (Heschl's gyrus), this may not be surprising. Symptom correlations have also been found with the hippocampus [40].

Schizophrenia as an active degenerative process

For many years it was thought that schizophrenia was not a degenerative disorder, but was rather more of a static encephalopathy [41], reflecting a primary neurodevelopmental pathology. In support of this, a number of studies have reported abnormalities in brain structure very early in the course of the disease [11,12,16,31,42,43]. However, there is increasing evidence to suggest that there may be progressive changes in brain structure subsequent to the onset of psychosis. For example, cross-sectional studies have suggested that chronic schizophrenics exhibit more severe structural abnormalities than first-episode patients in regions such as the hippocampus [43,44].

Longitudinal studies are required to resolve this issue of static versus progressive. A 4-year follow-up study of first-episode patients reported that they showed reduced left and right hemisphere volume, reduced volume of the right cerebellar hemisphere and increased left ventricular volume over time [42,45,46]. However, in contrast to the cross-sectional studies described above, no progressive reduction in hippocampal volume was observed in the schizophrenics as compared with controls. The authors argue that a 'subtle active brain process' is at work during the early years of the illness. Another longitudinal study obtained baseline and follow-up scans (on average 2.5 years later) of schizophrenics and controls, and reported longitudinal reduction in frontal lobe volume in patients compared with controls, also supporting the notion of a progressive disease process.

Some authors have attempted to integrate these two conflicting perspectives into a progressive neurodevelopmental model [47]. However, it is possible that progressive structural change only occurs in a subgroup of patients. In support of this, two longitudinal studies of ventricular volume showed that increased volume only occurred in a subset of subjects [7,48]. It is possible that different symptom clusters reflect different underlying cerebral changes [49], such that, for example, structural differences exist between patients with a positive history of auditory hallucinations compared with those without such a history. Such subgroups might display different disease progression in terms of both clinical state and brain structure. Were this to be true, it might help to explain some of the inconsistencies in the structural imaging literature.

The question of static or progressive is not purely of theoretical interest. If there is — in at least a subgroup of schizophrenics — progressive brain degeneration, then this holds out the possibility that such a disease process may be preventable with appropriate treatment.

Medication and brain structure

This idea of a link between antipsychotic medication and brain structure has become increasingly important in schizophrenia research. Although at first glance it might seem unlikely that drugs could produce measurable changes in regional brain volumes, there is a growing body of evidence to suggest that this is the case. An early study reported that, compared with controls, first-episode patients treated with typical neuroleptics had significantly increased caudate volume at 18 months' follow-up [50]. A follow-up study showed that a subset of the original sample of patients who were switched from typical drugs to clozapine showed a reduction in caudate volume at follow-up compared with those maintained on typical drugs [51]. Subsequent studies have confirmed this, showing that clozapine can reverse increases in caudate volume induced by typical neuroleptics [52], and that patients maintained on atypical drugs have reduced volumes of the caudate and putamen compared with those maintained on typical antipsychotics [53].

PET and SPECT studies (described in the next chapter) have shown that treatment with typical drugs leads to a very high level of striatal D_2 receptor blockade compared with clozapine which blocks fewer D_2 receptors. Therefore, the increase in basal ganglia volumes seen with typical drugs is probably due to their high level of D_2 receptor antagonism, which explains why clozapine with its lower D_2 blockade normalizes caudate volume. Differences in striatal D_2 receptor occupancy may explain the different rates of extrapyramidal side effects (EPS) seen with typical and atypical antipsychotic drugs.

Given the affinity of typical antipsychotic drugs for striatal D_2 receptors (see Chapter 4), it is not entirely surprising that medication effects have been observed here. To date, no one has demonstrated a medication effect on cortical regions. However, one study has suggested that this may be possible[33]. This study examined longitudinal change in the volume of the STG in drug-naive first-episode patients. The authors reported that, at baseline, the patients had reduced STG volume compared with controls. At 1-year follow-up, a subset of patients showed an increase in STG volume back towards that of controls. The cause of this increase is unclear, and there is no direct evidence that it is a medication effect. However, given the links between the STG and positive symptoms of psychotic illness[38], this tentative finding of possible reversibility of structural abnormalities is very exciting.

Brain structure and treatment response

A proportion of schizophrenics do not respond to typical neuroleptics but do improve on atypical drugs, while there is a significant minority of patients whose symptoms are resistant to every current pharmacological treatment, including clozapine. Given that early treatment of schizophrenia is increasingly realized to be important in terms of long-term prognosis, the ability to predict which patients will respond to which medications would make a huge difference to psychiatric practice. One growing area of research is the use of neuroimaging to find structural predictors of treatment response.

A study of patients during their first psychotic episode investigated the links between brain structure on MRI and the response to haloperidol[16]. It showed that the response to haloperidol was positively related to the total cortical grey matter, i.e. more grey matter was associated with a greater treatment response. In addition, increased cortical grey matter volume was associated with a lower dose needed to produce symptom improvement. Other studies have examined whether brain structure is related to patient response to clozapine, and have shown that enlargement of frontal[57] and temporal lobe sulci[55,56] is associated with a poorer response to clozapine.

Although these findings are interesting, until studies directly compare the response to different drugs in terms of brain anatomy, brain structure will have little predictive value in terms of guiding appropriate treatment.

Schizophrenia as a disorder of structural dysconnectivity

Given the number of brain structures that have been reported to be abnormal in schizophrenia, it is becoming increasingly clear that lesion models based on dysfunction in one structure or region are not accurate. Instead, research is beginning to consider schizophrenia as a disorder resulting from abnormal connections between different regions and structures.

The simplest method for testing for structural dysconnectivity is to examine correlations between the volumes of brain regions, to see whether they differ between patients and controls. Using this method, abnormalities in the connections between frontal and temporal lobe structures have been demonstrated[30,57,58], suggesting some type of fronto-temporal dysconnectivity[59], and between the frontal lobes and the thalamus [60]. A number of studies have examined the thalamus in schizophrenics [61], as it is densely connected with cortical regions, and it has been proposed that schizophrenic symptoms may arise from abnormalities in the connections between the frontal lobes, the thalamus and the cerebellum [62].

Interest in structural dysconnectivity has led to study of cerebral white matter changes, as white matter consists primarily of axonal bundles connecting cortical and subcortical regions. There is evidence of abnormalities in the size and shape of the corpus callosum (a structure consisting of bundles of white matter tracts connecting the two cerebral hemispheres), suggesting that interhemispheric connectivity may be abnormal in schizophrenia [63,64]. Studies of white matter volume have been contradictory, with some studies of chronic schizophrenia finding global and regional abnormalities [36,65,66], while others have found no difference, particularly in first-episode patients [16,67].

Although these findings strongly indicate abnormal structural connectivity in schizophrenia, they do not constitute definitive proof. Technological advances have seen the development of two techniques that permit direct assessment of fibre tracts connecting brain regions. Diffusion-weighted imaging (DWI) is a technique that allows for the assessment of the integrity and directionality of axonal bundles. A recent study using structural (DWI) and functional (PET) imaging showed that schizophrenic patients exhibited reduced diffusion anisotropy in the bundles connecting frontal and striatal regions, indicating abnormalities in the axonal bundles, and reduced correlations between frontal and striatal metabolic rate, providing evidence of both structural and functional dysconnectivity [68]. Other studies employing DWI in schizophrenia have reported both widespread white matter changes, in terms of reduced diffusion anisotropy [69], and localized changes in the corpus callosum, possibly suggesting reduced fibre density [70]. The other technique for assessing fibre tract status is magnetization transfer imaging (MTI), a technique that is believed to be highly sensitive to changes in myelination and axonal loss. A recent study using MTI found bilateral changes in the temporal lobes of schizophrenics [71].

These findings strongly suggest that structural dysconnectivity between brain regions is present in schizophrenia. However, the challenge is to understand the functional consequences of these white matter changes, their time-course and whether they are affected by antipsychotic medication.

Schizophrenia and loss of cerebral asymmetries

One current view of schizophrenia is that it is directly linked to the evolutionary development of language [72]. Given that there is no evolutionary advantage of schizophrenia (in that it is characterized by reduced fecundity), it is argued that it must arise as an abnormality from some evolutionarily advantageous development. Based on the fact that many schizophrenic symptoms are strongly linked to language abnormalities, it is suggested that schizophrenia is linked to the genetic event that allowed the human brain to develop the capacity for language.

In most people — be they right-handed or left-handed — language is left-hemisphere dominant, although it involves functions localized to the nondominant hemisphere. This functional specialization is presumed to reflect the genetic event that led to the development of language. Functional independence is paralleled by structural independence. Left-hemisphere specialization for language is reflected in left-right asymmetries in structures involved in language. This theory argues that there is a failure of lateralization of language in schizophrenia, and that this is manifested by a lack of normal hemispheric asymmetries in structures involved in language, and abnormal connections between them, i.e. abnormalities in the corpus callosum [64]. The most studied asymmetry in schizophrenia research has been the planum temporale (PT), a region on the posterior superior portion of the superior temporal gyrus that is heavily involved in language function [73]. In right-handed controls, the PT exhibits a normal left-larger-than-right asymmetry. However, a number of studies have provided evidence of loss or reversal of this asymmetry in schizophrenia — some studies have examined the surface area of the PT and reported a loss of normal left-larger-than-right asymmetry [74], while others have examined underlying grey matter and reported left PT grey matter loss [73]. Similarly, two recent studies have examined the inferior parietal lobe, a region that together with the PT is heavily involved in language functioning. Both studies showed that the normal pattern of left-larger-than-right volume asymmetry in controls was reversed in schizophrenics [75,76].

In addition to asymmetries in brain regions involved in language, other cerebral asymmetries have been studied in schizophrenia. The two cerebral hemispheres are normally highly asymmetric [77], with the right frontal lobe larger than the left, and the left occipital lobe larger than the right [78]. There is some evidence to suggest that these asymmetries are lost or even reversed in schizophrenia [79,80], and that these asymmetries are under genetic control [81].

However, this theory is not without problems. Firstly, structural asymmetries are much stronger in men than in women, and the majority of evidence for loss of asymmetries in schizophrenia is in males. Secondly, the theory assumes that there are genes in the human genome responsible for the development of cerebral asymmetries, and that these genes are abnormal in schizophrenia. However, thus far there is relatively little evidence for this.

High-dimensional brain mapping

Changes in the volumes of brain structures are a well-established finding in schizophrenia research. One new direction for the analysis of structural imaging data is high-dimensional brain mapping. This technique involves mapping one brain (or the average of a group) onto a template brain. It is possible to produce a variability map, indicating the areas of greatest difference between the new and the template brain (Figures 3–6). To do this, a computer program determines the extent to which the new brain has to be transformed into structural correspondence with the template. The following images demonstrate the level of detail that can be gleaned from this type of method compared with traditional volumetric methods.

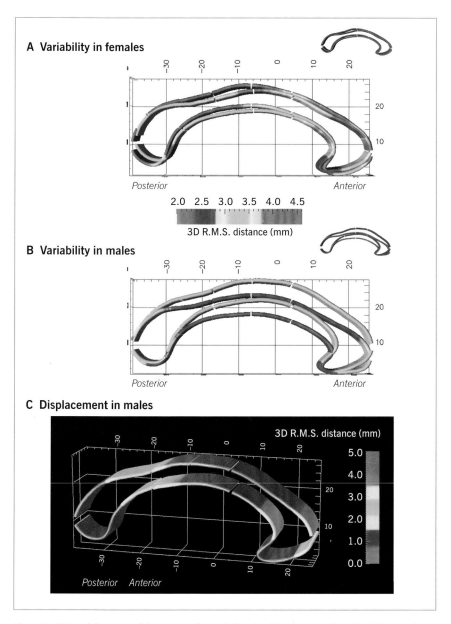

Figure 3. (A) Variability maps of the corpus callosum in female schizophrenic patients (dark-blue inset) and female controls (red inset). Average surface meshes reveal unique patterns of variability within each group. The colour bar encodes the root mean square magnitude (in millimetres) of the displacement vectors required to create the average callosum meshes. Female patients possess higher variability, especially in posterior regions, compared with female controls.

(B) Variability maps of the corpus callosum in male schizophrenic patients (dark-blue inset) and male controls (red inset). The corpus callosum appears more bowed in the vertical axis of the brain in male schizophrenic patients, reflecting a significant displacement in the inferior-superior direction as well as significant differences in callosal curvature across groups.

(C) Displacement between males only. This image shows the extent of regional difference between male schizophrenic patients and male controls.

Images courtesy of Katherine Narr and Dr Paul Thompson, Laboratory of Neuroimaging, UCLA. Narr KL, Thompson, PM, Sharma T et al. Mapping morphology of the corpus callosum in schizophrenia. Cereb Cortex 2000;**10***(1):40–90.*

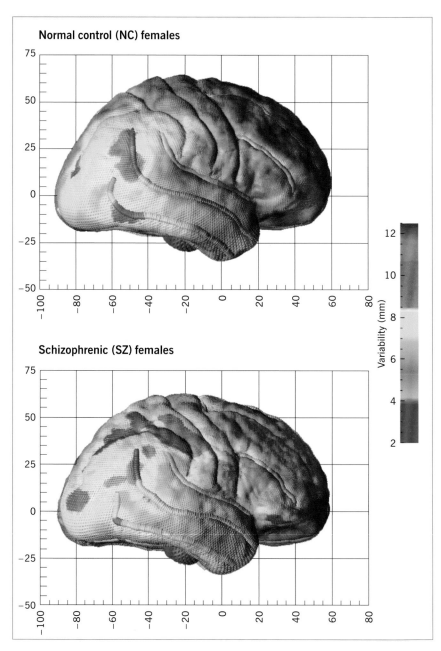

Figures 4 and 5. Variability maps of cortical surface and sulcal anatomy in normal controls (NC) and schizophrenic patients (SZ), showing the right hemisphere. The colour bar indicates patterns of variability in each group as the root mean square magnitude of displacement vectors from each point in the surface meshes. These maps show different profiles of sulcal variability in each group. Variability is increased at the superior limits of the superior temporal sulci in all groups. Increased variability is more apparent in the ascending ramus of the sylvian fissure in male groups, and higher in female groups for the ascending superior rami of the inferior temporal sulci. Overall, in both groups, maps of cortical surface variability seem to indicate increased individual differences in neopallial association areas in respect to phylogenetically and ontogenetically older areas of cortex.

Reproduced with permission from Narr KL, Sharma T, Moussai J et al. 3D maps of cortical surface variability and sulcal asymmetries in schizophrenic and normal populations. 5th International Conference on Functional Mapping of the Human Brain, *Dusseldorf, Germany, June 1999.*

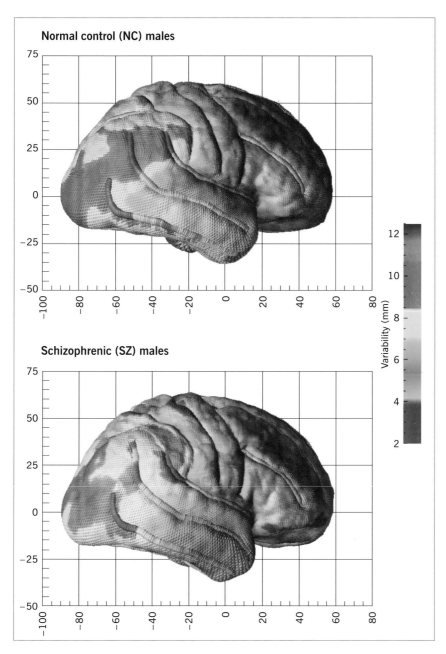

Figure 5. See legend on previous page.

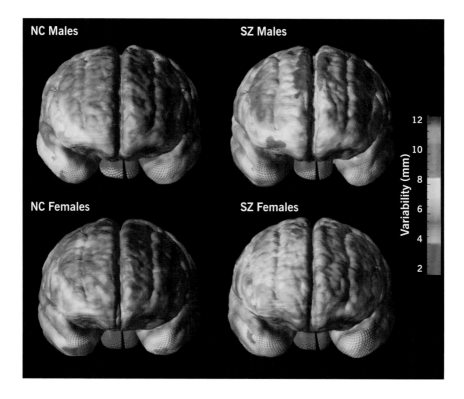

Figure 6. Cortical surface variability maps (front view) in the four groups defined by sex and diagnosis. The colour bar indicates patterns of variability within each group as the root mean square magnitude of displacement vectors required to map each individual onto the group average mesh. Increased variability is present in dorsolateral and orbitofrontal regions in schizophrenic patients.
Reproduced with permission from Narr KL, Sharma T, Moussai J et al. 3D maps of cortical surface variability and sulcal asymmetries in schizophrenic and normal populations. 5th International Conference on Functional Mapping of the Human Brain, *Dusseldorf, Germany, June 1999.*

This technique can be used to examine differences in cerebral morphometry (shape) between patient groups — such as schizophrenics or those with Alzheimer's disease — and controls[82]. The technique has already been used for analysis of structures such as the lateral ventricles[83] or corpus callosum in schizophrenia[63,84,85]. In a recent application of the method to the hippocampus in schizophrenia, it was shown that volumetric reductions in patients were due to abnormalities in the region of the hippocampus that projects to the prefrontal cortex[86]. Techniques are being developed that allow for automatic extraction of cortical and subcortical regions[87]. By going beyond simple volume comparisons, these and similar techniques will allow us to localize structural abnormalities more accurately, and to study much more subtle and microscopic changes.

Conclusions

CT and MRI studies have shown widespread structural abnormalities in schizophrenia, including ventricular enlargement and grey matter changes, suggesting widespread cortical malformation. However, for the most part, little is known about the clinical and cognitive consequences of these. The question of degenerative brain change remains to be resolved and is likely to have a significant impact on treatment, as would meaningful structural predictors of treatment response. New techniques such as DTI and MTI indicate diffuse changes in structural connectivity between brain regions, which require replication and clarification. High-dimensional mapping techniques should allow us better to characterize the structural abnormalities associated with this illness, together with providing an increased understanding of factors such as medication effects and illness chronicity.

References

1. Johnstone EC, Crow TJ, Frith CD et al. Cerebral ventricular size and cognitive impairment in chronic schizophrenia. *Lancet* 1976;**2**(7992):924–6.
2. Rossi A, Stratta P, de Cataldo S et al. Cortical and subcortical computed tomographic study in schizophrenia. *J Psychiatr Res* 1988;**22**:99–105.
3. Tanaka Y, Hazama H, Kawahara R et al. Computerized tomography of the brain in schizophrenic patients. A controlled study. *Acta Psychiatr Scand* 1981;**63**:191–7.
4. Weinberger DR, Cannon-Spoor E, Potkin SG et al. Poor premorbid adjustment and CT scan abnormalities in chronic schizophrenia. *Am J Psychiatry* 1980;**137**:1410–3.
5. Nasrallah HA, Kuperman S, Jacoby CG et al. Clinical correlates of sulcal widening in chronic schizophrenia. *Psychiatry Res (Neuroimaging)* 1983;**10**:237–42.
6. Kemali D, Maj M, Galderisi S et al. Clinical and neuropsychological correlates of cerebral ventricular enlargement in schizophrenia. *J Psychiatr Res* 1985;**19**:587–96.
7. Owen MJ, Lewis SW, Murray RM. Obstetric complications and schizophrenia: a computed tomographic study. *Psychol Med* 1988;**18**:331–9.
8. Takei N, Lewis S, Jones P et al. Prenatal exposure to influenza and increased cerebrospinal fluid spaces in schizophrenia. *Schizophr Bull* 1996;**22**:521–34.
9. Davis KL, Buchsbaum MS, Shihabuddin L et al. Ventricular enlargement in poor-outcome schizophrenia. *Biol Psychiatry* 1998;**43**:783–93.
10. Roy PD, Zipursky RB, Saint-Cyr JA et al. Temporal horn enlargement is present in schizophrenia and bipolar disorder. *Biol Psychiatry* 1998;**44**:418–22.
11. Nopoulos P, Torres I, Flaum M et al. Brain morphology in first-episode schizophrenia. *Am J Psychiatry* 1995;**152**:1721–3.
12. Lim KO, Tew W, Kushner M et al. Cortical gray matter volume deficit in patients with first-episode schizophrenia. *Am J Psychiatry* 1996;**153**:1548–53.
13. Sharma T, Lancaster E, Lee D et al. Brain changes in schizophrenia. Volumetric MRI study of families multiply affected with schizophrenia—the Maudsley Family Study 5. *Br J Psychiatry* 1998;**173**:132–8.
14. Lawrie SM, Abukmeil SS. Brain abnormality in schizophrenia. A systematic and quantitative review of volumetric magnetic resonance imaging studies. *Br J Psychiatry* 1998;**172**:110–20.
15. McCarley RW, Wible CG, Frumin M et al. MRI anatomy of schizophrenia. *Biol Psychiatry* 1999;**45**:1099–119.
16. Zipursky RB, Lambe EK, Kapur S et al. Cerebral gray matter volume deficits in first episode psychosis. *Arch Gen Psychiatry* 1998;**55**:540–6.
17. Gur RE, Turetsky BI, Bilker WB et al. Reduced gray matter volume in schizophrenia. *Arch Gen Psychiatry* 1999;**56**:905–11.
18. Wright IC, Rabe-Hesketh S, Woodruff PWR et al. Meta-analysis of regional brain volumes in schizophrenia. *Am J Psychiatry* 2000;**157**(1):16–25.
19. Buchanan RW, Vladar K, Barta PE et al. Structural evaluation of the prefrontal cortex in schizophrenia. *Am J Psychiatry* 1998;**155**:1049–55.
20. Wright IC, Ellison ZR, Sharma T et al. Mapping of grey matter changes in schizophrenia. *Schizophr Res* 1999;**35**:1–14.
21. Goldstein JM, Goodman JM, Seidman LJ et al. Cortical abnormalities in schizophrenia identified by magnetic resonance imaging. *Arch Gen Psychiatry* 1999;**56**:537–47.
22. Baare WF, Pol HE, Hijman R et al. Volumetric assessment of frontal lobe subregions in schizophrenia: relation to cognitive function and symptomatology. *Biol Psychiatry* 1999;**45**:1597–1605.

23. Wible CG, Shenton ME, Fischer IA et al. Parcellation of the human prefrontal cortex using MRI. *Psychiatry Res (Neuroimaging)* 1997;**76**:29–40.

24. Szeszko PR, Bilder RM, Lencz T et al. Investigation of frontal lobe subregions in first episode schizophrenia. *Psychiatry Res (Neuroimaging)* 1999;**90**:1–15.

25. Bogerts B, Meertz E, Schonfeldt-Bausch R. Basal ganglia and limbic system pathology in schizophrenia. A morphometric study of brain volume and shrinkage. *Arch General Psychiatry* 1985;**42**:784–91.

26. Bryant NL, Buchanan RW, Vladar K et al. Gender differences in temporal lobe structures of patients with schizophrenia: a volumetric MRI study. *Am J Psychiatry* 1999;**156**:603–9.

27. Hirayasu Y, Shenton ME, Salisbury DF et al. Lower left temporal lobe MRI volumes in patients with first-episode schizophrenia compared with psychotic patients with first-episode affective disorder and normal subjects. *Am J Psychiatry* 1998;**155**:1384–91.

28. Nelson MD, Saykin AJ, Flashman LA et al. Hippocampal volume reduction in schizophrenia as assessed by magnetic resonance imaging: a meta-analytic study. *Arch Gen Psychiatry* 1998;**55**:433–40.

29. Marsh L, Harris D, Lim KO et al. Structural magnetic resonance imaging abnormalities in men with severe chronic schizophrenia and an early age at clinical onset. *Arch Gen Psychiatry* 1997;**54**:1104–12.

30. Woodruff PW, Wright IC, Shuriquie N et al. Structural brain abnormalities in male schizophrenics reflect fronto-temporal dissociation. *Psychol Med* 1997;**27**:1257–66.

31. Velakoulis D, Pantelis C, McGorry PD et al. Hippocampal volume in first-episode psychoses and chronic schizophrenia: a high-resolution magnetic resonance imaging study. *Arch Gen Psychiatry* 1999;**56**(2):133–41.

32. Whitworth AB, Honeder M, Kremser C et al. Hippocampal volume reduction in male schizophrenic patients. *Schizophr Res* 1998;**31**:73–81.

33. Keshavan MS, Haas GL, Kahn CE et al. Superior temporal gyrus and the course of early schizophrenia: progressive, static, or reversible? *J Psychiatr Res* 1998;**32**:161–7.

34. Pearlson GD, Barta PE, Powers RE et al. Ziskind-Somerfeld Research Award 1996. Medial and superior temporal gyral volumes and cerebral asymmetry in schizophrenia versus bipolar disorder. *Biol Psychiatry* 1997;**41**:1–14.

35. Frangou S, Sharma T, Sigmudsson T et al. The Maudsley Family Study. 4. Normal planum temporale asymmetry in familial schizophrenia. A volumetric MRI study. *Br J Psychiatry* 1997;**170**:328–33.

36. Simgundsson T, Suckling J, Maier M et al. Structural abnormalities in frontal, temporal and limbic regions and interconnecting white matter tracts in schizophrenia. *Am J Psychiatry*, in press.

37. Barta PE, Pearlson GD, Powers RE et al. Auditory hallucinations and smaller superior temporal gyral volume in schizophrenia. *Am J Psychiatry* 1990;**147**:1457–62.

38. Shenton ME, Kikinis R, Jolesz FA et al. Abnormalities of the left temporal lobe and thought disorder in schizophrenia. A quantitative magnetic resonance imaging study. *New Engl J Med* 1992;**327**:604–12.

39. Flaum M, O'Leary DS, Swayze VW, 2nd et al. Symptom dimensions and brain morphology in schizophrenia and related psychotic disorders. *J Psychiatr Res* 1995;**29**:261–76.

40. Chua SE, Wright IC, Poline JB et al. Grey matter correlates of syndromes in schizophrenia. A semi-automated analysis of structural magnetic resonance images. *Br J Psychiatry* 1997;**170**:406–10.

41. Egan MF, Weinberger DR. Neurobiology of schizophrenia. *Curr Opin Neurobiol* 1997;**7**:701–7.

42. DeLisi LE, Hoff AL, Schwartz JE et al. Brain morphology in first-episode schizophrenic-like psychotic patients: a quantitative magnetic resonance imaging study. *Biol Psychiatry* 1991;**29**:159–75.

43. Bilder RM, Wu H, Bogerts B et al. Absence of regional hemispheric volume asymmetries in first-episode schizophrenia. *Am J Psychiatry* 1994;**151**:1437–47.

44. Razi K, Greene KP, Sakuma M, et al. Reduction of the parahippocampal gyrus and the hippocampus in patients with chronic schizophrenia. *Br J Psychiatry* 1999; **174**:512-519.

45. DeLisi LE, Tew W, Xie S et al. A prospective follow-up study of brain morphology and cognition in first-episode schizophrenic patients: preliminary findings. *Biol Psychiatry* 1995;**38**:349–60.

46. DeLisi LE, Sakuma M, Tew W et al. Schizophrenia as a chronic active brain process: a study of progressive brain structural change subsequent to the onset of schizophrenia. *Psychiatry Res* 1997;**74**:129–40.

47. Woods BT. Is schizophrenia a progressive neurodevelopmental disorder? Toward a unitary pathogenetic mechanism. *Am J Psychiatry* 1998;**155**:1661–70.

48. Nair TR, Christensen JD, Kingsbury SJ et al. Progression of cerebroventricular enlargement and the subtyping of schizophrenia. *Psychiatry Res* 1997;**74**:141–50.
49. Buchanan RW, Carpenter WT, Jr. The neuroanatomies of schizophrenia. *Schizophr Bull* 1997;**23**:367–72.
50. Chakos MH, Lieberman JA, Bilder RM et al. Increase in caudate nuclei volumes of first-episode schizophrenic patients taking antipsychotic drugs. *Am J Psychiatry* 1994;**151**:1430–6.
51. Chakos MH, Lieberman JA, Alvir J et al. Caudate nuclei volumes in schizophrenic patients treated with typical antipsychotics or clozapine. *Lancet* 1995;**345**:456–7.
52. Frazier JA, Giedd JN, Kaysen D et al. Childhood-onset schizophrenia: brain MRI rescan after 2 years of clozapine maintenance treatment. *Am J Psychiatry* 1996;**153**:564–6.
53. Corson PW, Nopoulos P, Miller DD et al. Change in basal ganglia volume over 2 years in patients with schizophrenia: typical versus atypical neuroleptics. *Am J Psychiatry* 1999;**156**(8):1200–4.
54. Friedman L, Knutson L, Shurell M et al. Prefrontal sulcal prominence is inversely related to response to clozapine in schizophrenia. *Biol Psychiatry* 1991;**29**:865–77.
55. Honer WG, Smith GN, Lapointe JS et al. Regional cortical anatomy and clozapine response in refractory schizophrenia. *Neuropsychopharmacology* 1995;**13**:85–7.
56. Lauriello J, Mathalon DH, Rosenbloom M et al. Association between regional brain volumes and clozapine response in schizophrenia. *Biol Psychiatry* 1998;**43**:879–86.
57. Wible CG, Shenton ME, Hokama H et al. Prefrontal cortex and schizophrenia. A quantitative magnetic resonance imaging study. *Arch Gen Psychiatry* 1995;**52**(4):279–88.
58. Bullmore ET, Woodruff PW, Wright IC et al. Does dysplasia cause anatomical dysconnectivity in schizophrenia? *Schizophr Res* 1998;**30**:127–35.
59. Fletcher P, McKenna PJ, friston KJ et al. Abnormal cingulate modulation of fronto-temporal connectivity in schizophrenia. *Neuroimage* 1999;**9**(3):337–42.
60. Portas CM, Goldstein JM, Shenton ME et al. Volumetric evaluation of the thalamus in schizophrenic male patients using magnetic resonance imaging. *Biol Psychiatry* 1998;**43**:649–59.
61. Andreasen NC, Arndt S, Swayze V et al. Thalamic abnormalities in schizophrenia visualized through magnetic resonance image averaging. *Science* 1994;**266**:294–8.
62. Andreasen NC, Paradiso S, O'Leary DS. "Cognitive dysmetria" as an integrative theory of schizophrenia: a dysfunction in cortical-subcortical-cerebellar circuitry? *Schizophr Bull* 1998;**24**:203–18.
63. Narr KL, Thompson PM, Sharma T et al. Mapping morphology of the corpus callosum in schizophrenia. *Cereb Cortex* 2000;**10**(1):40–9.
64. Crow TJ. Schizophrenia as a transcallosal misconnection syndrome. *Schizophr Res* 1998;**30**:111–4.
65. Buchanan RW, Vladar K, Barta PE et al. Structural evaluation of the prefrontal cortex in schizophrenia. *Am J Psychiatry* 1998;**155**:1049–55.
66. Cannon TD van Erp TG, Huttunen M et al. Regional gray matter, white matter, and cerebrospinal fluid distributions in schizophrenic patients, their siblings, and controls. *Arch Gen Psychiatry* 1998;**55**:1084–91.
67. Lim KO, Tew W, Kushner M et al. Cortical gray matter volume deficit in patients with first-episode schizophrenia. *Am J Psychiatry* 1996;**153**:1548–53.
68. Buchsbaum MS, Tang CY, Peled S et al. MRI white matter diffusion anisotropy and PET metabolic rate in schizophrenia. *Neuroreport* 1998;**9**:425–30.
69. Lim KO, Hedehus M, Moseley M et al. Compromised white matter tract integrity inferred from diffusion tensor imaging. *Arch Gen Psychiatry* 1999;**56**:367–74.
70. Foong J, Maier M, Barker GJ et al. In vivo investigation of white matter pathology in schizophrenia with magnetisation transfer imaging. *J Neurol Neurosurg Psychiatry* 2000;**68**:70–4.
71. Foong J, Maier M, Clark CA et al. Neuropathological abnormalities of the corpus callosum in schizophrenia: a diffusion tensor imaging study. *J Neurol Neurosurg Psychiatry* 2000;**68**:242–4.
72. Crow TJ. Is schizophrenia the price that Homo sapiens pays for language? *Schizophr Res* 1997;**28**:127–41.
73. Kwon JS, McCarley RW, Hirayasu Y et al. Left planum temporale volume reduction in schizophrenia. *Arch Gen Psychiatry* 1999;**56**:142–8.
74. Barta PE, Pearlson GD, Brill LB et al. Planum temporale asymmetry reversal in schizophrenia: replication and relationship to gray matter abnormalities. *Am J Psychiatry* 1997;**154**:661–7.
75. Niznikiewicz M, Donnino R, McCarley RW et al. Abnormal angular gyrus asymmetry in schizophrenia. *Am J Psychiatry* 2000;**157**:428–37.

76. Frederikse M, Lu A, Aylward E et al. Sex differences in inferior parietal lobule volume in schizophrenia. *Am J Psychiatry* 2000;**157**:422–7.

77. Petty RG. Structural asymmetries of the human brain and their disturbance in schizophrenia. *Schizophr Bull* 1999;**25**:121–39.

78. Bilder RM, Wu H, Bogerts B et al. Absence of regional hemispheric volume asymmetries in first-episode schizophrenia. *Am J Psychiatry* 1994;**151**:1437–47.

79. Sharma T, Lancaster E, Sigmundsson T, et al. Lack of normal pattern of cerebral asymmetry in familial schizophrenic patients and their relatives – The Maudsley Family Study. *Schizophr Res* 1999; **40(2)**:111-120.

80. Bilder RM, Wu H, Bogerts B et al. Cerebral volume asymmetries in schizophrenia and mood disorders: a quantitative magnetic resonance imaging study. *Int J Psychophysiol* 1999;**34**:197–205.

81. Thompson PM, Moussai J, Zohoori S et al. Cortical variability and asymmetry in normal aging and Alzheimer's disease. *Cereb Cortex* 1998;**8**:492–509.

82. Buckley PF, Dean D, Bookstein FL et al. Three-dimensional magnetic resonance-based morphometrics and ventricular dysmorphology in schizophrenia. *Biol Psychiatry* 1999;**45**:62–7.

83. Tibbo P, Nopoulos P, Arndt S et al. Corpus callosum shape and size in male patients with schizophrenia. *Biol Psychiatry* 1998;**44**:405–12.

84. DeQuardo JR, Keshavan MS, Bookstein FL et al. Landmark-based morphometric analysis of first-episode schizophrenia. *Biol Psychiatry* 1999;**45**:1321–8.

85. Csernansky JG, Joshi S, Wang L et al. Hippocampal morphometry in schizophrenia by high dimensional brain mapping. *Proc Natl Acad Sci USA* 1998;**95**:11406–11.

86. Le Goualher G, Proyck E, Collins DL et al. Automated extraction and variability analysis of sulcal neuroanatomy. *IEEE Trans Med Imaging* 1999;**18**:206–17.

87. Zhou Y, Thompson PM, Toga AW. Extracting and representing the cortical sulci. *IEEE Computer Graphics and Applications* 1999;**19**:49–55.

CHAPTER 4
Functional Brain Imaging in Schizophrenia

Understanding how the structure of the brain may be abnormal in schizophrenia has been central to advancing our knowledge of the illness. However, possibly the most exciting advances in schizophrenia research have followed from neuroimaging techniques that facilitate the visualization of brain function. These allow us to investigate, at a global and regional level, the neurochemical and neurovascular systems that may be abnormal in schizophrenia. This offers the potential to understand how functional changes may link to the cognitive dysfunction and primary symptoms of schizophrenia, and how these may be affected by antipsychotic medication.

PET and SPECT imaging of neurotransmitter receptors

The development of in vivo neuroimaging techniques such as positron emission tomography (PET) and single photon emission computed tomography (SPECT) has greatly advanced research into the neurobiology and treatment of schizophrenia. PET and SPECT studies of receptor occupancy are helping to answer questions relating to the activity of potentially abnormal neurochemical systems, and the mechanism of action of different antipsychotic drugs.

Early theories of neurochemical dysfunction in schizophrenia focused on the dopamine system as a potential site of abnormality, and therefore a possible treatment target [1]. In support of this, there is evidence that all antipsychotic medications strongly block mesolimbic dopamine receptors. For example, in an early study, Farde et al. demonstrated a high level of striatal dopamine D_2 receptor occupancy in medicated schizophrenics compared with controls [2]. Bigliani et al. [3] showed that patients treated with typical antipsychotics showed high levels of D_2 and D_3 receptor antagonism in the striatum and in temporal lobe regions, while Kapur et al. [4] found a relationship between striatal D_2 receptor blockade and positive symptom improvement. Given the known efficacy of typical drugs in treating the positive symptoms of psychosis, these studies suggest that dopaminergic receptor blockade is likely to mediate the antipsychotic properties of these drugs.

Although typical antipsychotics are very good at treating positive psychotic symptoms, they have little effect on negative symptoms and cognitive function, and are also associated with a higher incidence of extrapyramidal side effects (EPS). Conversely, atypical antipsychotic drugs are associated with greater efficacy in treating negative symptoms, improvements in cognitive functioning and a lower rate of EPS [5]. Therefore many studies have compared the receptor binding profiles of typical and atypical antipsychotics, in the hope of identifying the pharmacological mechanisms that underpin these differences.

Some studies have compared the activity of typical and atypical drugs at dopamine receptors. For example, Broich et al. [6] compared clozapine-treated, typically-treated

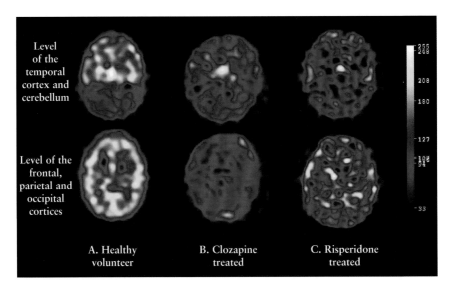

Figure 1. ^{123}I-5-I-R91150 SPECT brain scan of 5-HT$_{2A}$ receptors. (A) Healthy volunteer on no medication. (B) Volunteer with schizophrenia treated with clozapine 450 mg per day. (C) Volunteer with schizophrenia treated with risperidone 6 mg per day.
Reproduced with permission from Travis et al. [8]

and medication-free schizophrenics in a SPECT study examining the links between D$_2$ receptor blockade and side effects [6]. Patients on typical neuroleptics were found to have a much higher level of striatal D$_2$ receptor blockade, and a higher incidence of EPS, compared with those who were drug free or on clozapine. Similarly, a SPECT study by Kasper et al. comparing three atypical drugs — clozapine, risperidone and sertindole — with haloperidol showed that haloperidol and high-dose risperidone (8 mg) both induced high levels of D$_2$ receptor occupancy (>70%), with clozapine inducing a 33% receptor blockade and sertindole blocking an intermediate 60% of receptors [7]. These results suggest that the mechanism of atypicality is not merely reduced D$_2$ receptor antagonism.

Consequently, research has begun to investigate the affinity of atypical drugs for other neurotransmitter receptors for an explanation of their atypicality. The realization that atypical drugs bind strongly to 5-HT (serotonin) receptors has sparked great interest in this neurotransmitter system as a potential site of antipsychotic action. Travis et al. used SPECT to study the extent to which clozapine and risperidone blocked 5-HT$_{2A}$ receptors [8]. The results showed no differences in receptor occupancy between clozapine- and risperidone-treated patients, indicating a high degree of 5-HT$_{2A}$ receptor blockade with both drugs (Figure 1).

In a recent series of PET studies, Kapur and colleagues studied the dopamine and 5-HT receptor binding characteristics of several antipsychotic drugs, and the relationship between receptor occupancy, symptoms and side-effects. Kapur et al. investigated the degree of D$_2$ and 5-HT$_2$ receptor blockade induced by different doses of the atypical drug olanzapine, and how these related to clinical efficacy and side-effects [9]. Even at small doses (5 mg), the drug blocked virtually all cortical

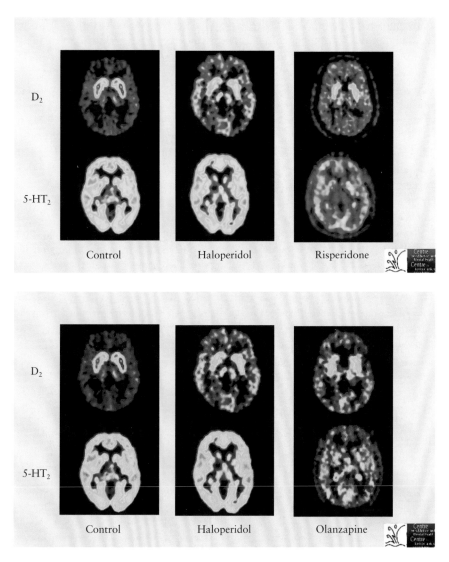

Figure 2. PET images of D_2 and 5-HT_2 receptor occupancy in healthy controls and schizophrenics on different antipsychotic medications. Brighter regions indicate a high degree of ligand binding (and therefore low drug-induced receptor blockade). Compared to haloperidol, both olanzapine and risperidone block many more cortical 5-HT_2 receptors, while all three drugs block striatal D_2 receptors.
Images courtesy of Dr Shitij Kapur, Schizophrenia Division, Clarke Institute, Toronto, Canada.

5-HT_2 receptors. D_2 receptor occupancy was related to dose, with 55% striatal D_2 occupancy at 5 mg daily, rising to 88% occupancy with doses of 40 mg. Interestingly, two patients who did not respond to low-dose (5 or 10 mg) olanzapine still did not respond at doses of 30 or 40 mg, despite a significant rise in striatal D_2 receptor antagonism. Subsequently, Kapur et al. compared the D_2 and 5-HT_2 occupancy of clozapine, olanzapine and risperidone [5]. Consistent with other studies, all three drugs exhibited a higher level of 5-HT_2 than D_2 receptor occupancy, while risperidone (5 mg) and olanzapine (20 mg) showed high levels of D_2 antagonism, similar to low dose typical antipsychotics, and clozapine blocked fewer dopamine receptors. In their study of haloperidol-treated patients, Kapur et al. found a relationship not only between D_2 receptor occupancy and clinical improvement, but also with incidence of EPS [4]. A moderate degree (60%+) of D_2 blockade was sufficient to begin to see clinical change, while side-effects began to develop with occupancy above about 80%. Figure 2 shows example PET images of the different binding patterns of typical and atypical antipsychotics to D_2 and $5\text{-}HT_2$ receptors.

It is clear from all these studies that most atypical antipsychotic drugs do not induce substantially lower blockade of dopamine receptors than do typical agents. They suggest that while high levels of EPS seen with treatment with typical antipsychotic drugs may be due to high levels of striatal D_2 receptor blockade, the lower incidence in patients treated with atypical medications is not due to lower levels of D_2 receptor occupancy. One alternative possibility is that high levels of $5\text{-}HT_2$ receptor antagonism protect against the development of these side-effects. In support of this idea, Kapur et al. [10] and Nyberg et al. [11] compared the dopamine receptor occupancy of different doses of risperidone and showed that increasing dose was associated with increased receptor occupancy and a greater risk of developing EPS. Kapur et al. suggested that 5-HT receptor blockade may provide a "relative protection" from the development of EPS, such that this protection is lost at very high levels of D_2 receptor blockade. This would explain how increasing dosages of atypical drugs are associated with a higher incidence of EPS.

Clozapine, often termed the prototypical atypical antipsychotic drug, appears to be unique in terms of its mechanism of action, with low D_2 and high 5-HT receptor blockade. High levels of 5-HT receptor occupancy seen with clozapine and other atypical antipsychotic drugs may explain the improvements in negative symptomatology and cognition that are associated with their use [5]. However, it is important to note that very few of these studies have found a link between the extent of dopamine or 5-HT receptor binding and measures of symptomatology. This suggests that schizophrenia is not a simple abnormality in one neurotransmitter system, but rather may reflect a more widespread neurochemical disturbance, possibly involving abnormal modulation of various transmitter systems. New ligands are constantly being developed that will enable researchers to study other dopamine and serotonin receptor subtypes, as well as neurotransmitters such as glutamate and noradrenaline. Understanding the complex interactions between these systems should aid in the development of better targeted drugs.

PET, SPECT and fMRI of brain activity

In addition to studying neurotransmitter systems, there has been extensive interest in studying cerebral activity in schizophrenia. PET and SPECT studies have examined glucose metabolism and regional blood flow (rCBF), while more recently research has begun to capitalise on the spatial and temporal superiority offered by functional magnetic resonance imaging (fMRI). Using these approaches, functional imaging studies have examined links between brain activation, cognitive functioning and symptoms, in the hope of identifying those regions and circuits that may be abnormal in schizophrenia.

Symptoms and brain activity – PET and SPECT

Recent research has examined whether the major symptoms of schizophrenia can be linked to abnormal functioning of one or more brain regions. Answering this question may help to identify where antipsychotic drugs should be targeted.

In a landmark paper, Liddle et al. investigated the links between patterns of rCBF and schizophrenic symptoms [12]. They identified three primary symptom clusters — psychomotor poverty, disorganization and reality distortion — and examined whether these were characterized by different patterns of cerebral perfusion. The results showed that reality distortion scores were positively correlated with blood flow in the hippocampal region and the left prefrontal cortex. Patient scores on the disorganization factor were associated with reduced blood flow in the right prefrontal cortex, together with reduced activity of a left temporal lobe region involved in speech production. Lastly, psychomotor poverty was characterized by reduced activity in the left dorsolateral prefrontal cortex and anterior cingulate. This finding provided support for the idea that negative symptoms are characterized by frontal lobe dysfunction. Other studies have reported similar findings [13,14,16]. Reduced activity in prefrontal regions as seen in the Liddle et al. study is termed *hypofrontality*, and, as shall be seen below, has become a central theme in functional imaging research [12].

A number of studies have suggested that some positive symptoms of schizophrenia, such as hallucinations, delusions and thought disorder, are associated with abnormal activity of frontal and temporal lobe structures involved in language. McGuire et al. studied a group of schizophrenics both while they were experiencing hallucinations and later when their symptoms had remitted [15]. Using SPECT, the hallucinatory state in the patients was characterized by increased blood in the left inferior frontal cortex (which contains Broca's area), left temporal lobe and anterior cingulate. McGuire et al. compared schizophrenics who had a history of auditory hallucinations with non-hallucinators, and observed that, when asked to imagine another person speaking a sentence, the hallucinators failed to activate temporal and frontal regions — both of which regions were activated by non-hallucinators and controls [18]. In another study, McGuire et al. investigated rCBF when psychotic subjects were producing thought-disordered speech in response to pictures [19]. The results showed that thought-disordered speech was positively correlated with blood flow in the parahippocampal region and the right caudate nucleus. Thought disorder was negatively correlated with blood flow in the left and right inferior frontal gyri, left superior temporal gyrus and cingulate gyrus, again implicating abnormal activation of language areas of the brain.

Symptoms and brain activity – fMRI

fMRI has also been used to study the link between regional cerebral activation and psychotic symptoms. Woodruff et al. used fMRI to investigate brain regions that might be important in auditory hallucinations [20]. As in the studies described earlier, these workers compared a group of schizophrenic patients who had a history of hallucinations with a group who had no such history. Additionally, a group of patients were scanned both while experiencing hallucinations and again when their symptoms had reduced. All subjects were asked to listen to a tape of someone speaking. The results showed that while healthy controls showed major increases in activity in left temporal regions, schizophrenics showed less functional lateralization, with an increase in right middle temporal gyrus activity. A comparison of schizophrenics when hallucinating and when in remission showed that the hallucinatory state was associated with reduced activity in the right middle temporal gyrus and the left superior temporal gyrus. Given that the right middle temporal gyrus is normally activated by external speech, reduced activation might result in abnormal speech and thought perception. Functional abnormalities in the superior temporal gyrus parallel reported structural abnormalities [21]. Recently, Dierk et al. performed fMRI studies in schizophrenics who were hallucinating and again when they were not, and found that hallucinations were associated with increased activity in Heschl's gyrus, a temporal lobe region containing the primary auditory cortex [22].

The results from all these PET, SPECT and fMRI studies support the notion of abnormal activity of language- and speech-related areas of the brain in schizophrenia. As an explanation of these findings, it has been suggested that symptoms such as auditory hallucinations are due to a failure of self-monitoring [17], such that inner speech (thinking in words) is not recognized as such, but instead is perceived as 'alien' [18].

Symptoms and brain activity – state or trait?

Are abnormalities in brain activation in schizophrenia, such as hypofrontality, relatively stable phenomena, or are they more closely linked to illness severity? Several studies described above involved longitudinal scanning of patients when acutely ill and when their symptoms had remitted [15,20]. They showed that patterns of brain activity differed markedly between the florid and remitted states. Similarly, Spence et al. carried out repeat PET scans in a group of patients during an acute phase and again when they were in remission [23]. Results showed that during a motor activation task, patients had reduced activity of the dorsolateral prefrontal cortex at baseline (when psychotic), but that they showed increased blood flow in this region 4–6 weeks later when their symptoms were improving. This finding has subsequently been replicated by Erkwoh et al. who found, using SPECT, that remission of active symptoms was associated with increased rCBF in frontal and temporal regions [24]. These studies suggest that features such as hypofrontality and abnormal activation of temporal cortical regions represent state rather than trait phenomena. This work has exciting implications for the study of brain function in schizophrenia.

Brain imaging and cognition – PET and SPECT

The notion of hypofrontality described above has become a central theme of functional imaging research in schizophrenia. The original study by Ingvar and Franzen [25] was followed by a large number of resting-state studies suggesting reduced frontal activity [26], probably linked to negative symptoms [13]. Subsequently, studies have moved on from resting-state assessment to examine cerebral blood flow during performance of a cognitive task. Although the literature is very contradictory, there is evidence to show that hypofrontality in schizophrenia is not merely a resting-state phenomenon, but is also reflected in reduced activation of frontal regions during task performance [27,28].

For example, an early PET study looked at brain activity in schizophrenics during performance of the Wisconsin Card Sorting Test (WCST), a test of executive function believed to test prefrontal cortical functioning [29]. This study showed that, while performing the WCST, patients exhibited significantly less activation in the dorsolateral prefrontal cortex than did controls. Similarly, a SPECT study by Andreasen et al. used another test of prefrontal functioning, the Tower of London paradigm, and found decreased activation of the left prefrontal cortex, but only in patients with predominantly negative symptoms [27].

It should be pointed out that changes in brain activation are not limited to frontal regions. For example, a recent study identified functional changes in episodic memory function in schizophrenia [30]. This study compared brain activity in schizophrenics and controls while recollecting previously studied words, and showed that, compared to controls, schizophrenics showed normal activation of the dorsolateral prefrontal cortex, but reduced activation of the hippocampus. In a subsequent study, it was shown that, during memory retrieval, patients with mainly negative symptoms exhibited reduced prefrontal activation compared to patients without negative symptoms, again supporting the argument that hypofrontality is related to negative symptomatology [31].

Brain imaging and cognition – fMRI

Volz et al. used fMRI to examine regional brain activation during performance of the WCST in patients with schizophrenia [32]. Results showed that the schizophrenics made significantly more errors than the controls, and exhibited significantly less activation of the right prefrontal cortex, together with increased activation of left temporal regions. This is consistent with previous PET studies of hypofrontality in schizophrenia. The authors suggest that increased left temporal lobe activity may reflect 'abnormal cerebral co-ordination' of activity between brain regions.

Another domain where schizophrenics often show impairment is working memory, which has major implications for normal daily functioning. Stevens et al. found that, whereas controls showed increased activity in the left inferior frontal gyrus during both verbal and non-verbal working memory tasks, this activation was greatly reduced in schizophrenics [33]. Reduced activation was also observed in some temporal lobe regions. Together with the findings of structural abnormalities in the inferior prefrontal cortex, these results strongly implicate this region in the cognitive deficits and symptoms associated with schizophrenia [34].

Studies have shown that brain activity during tasks such as verbal fluency is abnormal in schizophrenics [35]. In a study exploring this further, Curtis et al. found that chronic schizophrenics showed reduced activity in the left middle and inferior frontal gyri during a word-generation task, and increased activation in parietal regions during a word-repetition task, compared with control subjects (Figure 4) [36].

Curtis et al. went on to investigate the extent to which hypofrontality may be a task-specific phenomenon [37]. Having observed hypofrontality with verbal fluency, they investigated patterns of regional activation during a semantic decision task. The results showed that, compared with controls, the schizophrenics did not exhibit

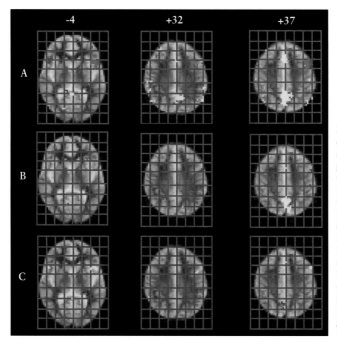

Figure 4. Patterns of cerebral activation during word generation (red) and word repetition (yellow). (A) Areas of increased activation in controls. (B) Areas of increased activity in schizophrenics. (C) Regions where significant differences in activity were observed between patients and controls. *Reproduced with permission from Curtis et al.* [36]

hypofrontality; however, they did demonstrate an abnormal pattern of brain activation, with higher levels of activity bilaterally in the fusiform and lingual gyri, and in the right inferior temporal gyri (Figure 5). The results of these fMRI studies suggest that changes in brain activity in schizophrenia are widespread and more complex than simply reduced activity in prefrontal regions.

Schizophrenia as a disorder of functional connectivity

In a similar way to some of the structural imaging studies described in Chapter 2, functional imaging research has moved away from looking at schizophrenia as resulting from abnormalities in one or two regions — a *lesion* model — to looking at changes in neural circuits. Most brain regions are highly interconnected, and most tasks recruit the involvement of spatially distributed structures. Several of the studies discussed above have reported abnormal activity in various regions in schizophrenics. Functional dysconnectivity implies that the normal pattern of distributed activation, and the relationship(s) between activation in regions, is abnormal.

Functional dysconnectivity may provide an explanation for many of the symptoms and cognitive deficits associated with schizophrenia. Indeed, Andreasen et al. concluded that distributed abnormalities in brain activity in schizophrenia reflect a number of dysfunctional circuits that result in "impairment of the ability to set priorities, process and produce information, and to turn it into meaningful thoughts and behaviour. This imbalance in circuits is expressed as psychotic or negative symptoms" [26]. Although there is relatively widespread agreement that functional connectivity is abnormal in schizophrenia, debate continues about which circuits are abnormal.

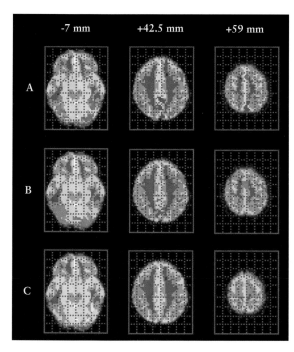

Figure 5. Patterns of cerebral activation during a semantic decision task. (A) Activity for control subjects. (B) Activity in schizophrenics. (C) Regions where significant differences in levels of activation were observed between patients and controls.
Reproduced with permission from Curtis et al. [37]

Wiser et al. used ^{15}O-labelled water to study rCBF during a memory task and reported that, despite equal task performance between patients and controls, the two groups activated different circuits to perform the task [38]. The patients were found to perform the task with significantly smaller increases in blood flow to the inferior, middle and medial frontal cortex, and left cerebellar cortex, compared with controls. Furthermore, patients showed increased blood flow to the anterior cingulate, right superior temporal gyrus and fusiform gyrus when compared with controls. Wiser and co-workers [38] argue that the reduced blood flow in the prefrontal cortex and the cerebellum supports the idea of cognitive dysmetria [39]. They define this as "a disruption of the interaction between cortical (especially frontal) functions such as initiation of memory retrieval or working memory, and cerebellar functions such as timing and sequencing, leading to cognitive misconnections and a disruption of the fluid co-ordination of mental activity." They argue that abnormalities in frontothalamic cerebellar circuits provide an explanation of both positive and negative symptoms.

An alternative view of functional dysconnectivity has come from a study by Jennings et al. using PET scanning of regional brain activity during a semantic processing task [40]. They employed a technique known as path analysis, with which it is possible to study how a change in activity in one region affects activity in the region to which it projects. Using this, Jennings and colleagues showed that regions that were positively connected in controls — i.e. increased activity in one led to increased activity in the other — were negatively connected in the schizophrenics. In particular, abnormalities were seen in connections between frontal and temporal regions, and between frontal regions and the anterior cingulate.

Abnormalities in connections between frontal and temporal regions and the cingulate have been supported by other studies. A recent study examined the functional relationship between the dorsolateral prefrontal cortex (DLPFC), superior temporal gyrus and cingulate during a memory task [41]. The authors hypothesised that abnormal activity in the superior temporal gyrus would be related to the relationship between activity in the DLPFC and cingulate. The results showed that, in controls, increased activity in the DLPFC and cingulate led to less activity in the STG, while in patients the pattern was reversed, such that increased activity in the cingulate and DPLFC was accompanied by a failure to deactivate the STG. The authors suggest that this reflects abnormal modulation by the cingulate of the effects of prefrontal cortical activity on the STG. In support of this type of dysconnectivity, another study reported abnormal connectivity between the left DLPFC and cingulate in a group of schizophrenics [42].

Other studies have reported evidence of an abnormal functional relationship between frontal and striatal regions. For example, Buchsbaum et al. looked at correlations between metabolic rates in the frontal lobes and the striatum, and showed that these correlations were significantly lower in schizophrenics than in controls [43]. Subsequently, in a study of drug-naive patients, a similar pattern of reduced correlations between frontal and striatal regions was observed [44].

It is clear that research into functional connectivity is in its infancy. A greater understanding of normal functional circuits is a necessary precursor of future disease-related work. It is currently unknown whether abnormal functional connectivity is a stable phenomenon, and how it relates to symptom state and medication.

Functional neuroimaging of drug effects

As has already been described, there is a large body of evidence regarding the different pharmacological profiles of typical and atypical antipsychotic drugs. However, relatively little is known about their differential effects on cerebral function. Studies are beginning to use functional imaging to study the effects of different antipsychotic drugs on cerebral activity. The ability to monitor the effects of antipsychotic drugs on brain activity is likely to aid greatly our understanding of how drugs work, and help us to identify which drug would be most suitable for a particular patient.

In Chapter 3, studies were discussed that showed that typical antipsychotic drugs were associated with increased volumes of basal ganglia structures [45]. One possible explanation for this is that it reflects increased blood flow in these structures. There is evidence from a PET study to support this idea [46]. The authors examined rCBF in a group of schizophrenics while they were on typical antipsychotics and subsequently after a three week drug-free period. The results showed that the schizophrenics exhibited higher blood flow in the basal ganglia when medicated, compared to their drug-free state, together with decreased rCBF in frontal lobe regions. This supports the notion that medication-induced structural changes in the basal ganglia may reflect vascular changes.

A recent fMRI study has suggested that antipsychotic medication may exert an influence on neuronal function in schizophrenics. Honey et al. studied whether

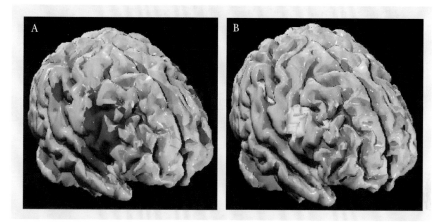

Figure 6. Rendered images of the brain showing regions of increased activity following substitution of risperidone for typical antipsychotics. (A) Brain activity related to memory. (B) Specific areas of improved brain function following treatment with risperidone.
Image courtesy of Garry Honey, Section of Cognitive Psychopharmacology, and John Suckling, Brain Image Analysis Unit, Institute of Psychiatry, London.

switching schizophrenics from typical antipsychotic drugs to the atypical drug risperidone would produce differences in brain activity during a working memory task [47]. Working memory deficits have been consistently reported in schizophrenia, and there is evidence of functional hypofrontality during working memory tasks [33]. Given that working memory performance has been shown to be related to prefrontal dopamine function [48], and that there is evidence from animal studies that atypical antipsychotics increase prefrontal dopamine transmission [49], the authors predicted that switching schizophrenics from typical antipsychotics to risperidone would result in increased activity of prefrontal regions.

Patients were scanned at a baseline assessment when treated with typical antipsychotic drugs. Subsequently half of the group were switched to risperidone while the other half remained on their typical medication. Subjects were rescanned after 6 weeks. The results showed that patients switched to risperidone exhibited an increase in blood oxygenation in the right DLPFC, precuneus and supplementary motor area (SMA) at follow-up (Figure 6). The authors observe that the cause of the observed increased frontal cortical activity may reflect the effect of reduced D_2 receptor antagonism, serotonin-induced reduced activity of inhibitory GABA neurones, or alternatively serotonin-mediated increased frontal dopamine activity.

This shows that it may be possible to 'reactivate' brain regions in psychiatric illness via drug treatment. The increased activation in prefrontal regions may help to explain the improvements in cognitive functioning that have been observed with risperidone [50]. This study also demonstrates the suitability of fMRI as a tool to assess psychopharmacological effects. Given that fMRI has many advantages for longitudinal study over techniques such as PET and SPECT, this sort of approach could be used to study drug effects in other psychiatric disorders, such as the effects of cholinesterase inhibitors in Alzheimer's Disease.

Magnetic resonance spectroscopy and schizophrenia

Magnetic resonance spectroscopy (MRS) is increasingly being used to investigate molecular abnormalities in schizophrenia in vivo, and how these may be linked to symptomatology and cognitive function.

MRS works on the same principles as MRI. A radio-frequency pulse applied to nuclei causes their magnetic moments to alter their orientation. When the pulse is switched off, the moments realign and give off a radio-frequency signal that can be detected. According to the local chemical environment, the nuclei give off a different frequency signal — this is known as the chemical shift phenomenon, and gives the different peaks seen on an MR spectrum. Kegeles et al. provide an excellent review of MRS and schizophrenia [51].

Spectroscopy of the frontal lobes

A large part of this chapter has been devoted to the discussion of prefrontal cortical dysfunction in schizophrenia [32,37]. MRS studies have also extensively investigated this region.

In an early study using ^{31}P spectroscopy, Pettergrew et al. investigated the dorsolateral prefrontal cortex of drug-naive and first-episode schizophrenic patients [52]. The spectral patterns obtained showed decreased levels of phosphomonoesters (PMEs) and inorganic phosphate (Pi), whilst levels of adenosine diphosphate (ADP) and phosphodiesters (PDEs) were elevated. Other studies of the dorsolateral prefrontal cortex have also reported decreased levels of PMEs [53]. Deicken et al. studied frontal and parietal regions, and reported increased levels of PDEs, together with decreased levels of phosphocreatine (PCr) and Pi [54]. In a recent study using proton-decoupled spectroscopy — which is capable of separating the contributing chemicals to spectroscopy signals — increases in frontal lobe PDE levels were observed to be due to increased levels of membrane-bound chemicals, rather than increased levels of membrane breakdown products [55]. Decreased levels of Pi and phosphocholine were also seen. Together, these findings in relation to PMEs and PDEs are suggestive of abnormal cell membrane structure and activity in prefrontal regions. As most energy consumption is related to neurotransmitter activity and related processes, changes in levels of energy-related chemicals such as ATP, PCr and Pi are indicative of abnormal neuronal activity.

Studies using proton spectroscopy have also found evidence of abnormal frontal lobe chemistry. Deicken et al. [56] reported lower levels of frontal lobe N-acetyl aspartate (NAA, a putative neuronal marker), as did Bertolino et al. [57,58], who also reported reduced ratios of NAA/choline (Cho) and NAA/creatine (Cr) levels in the dorsolateral prefrontal cortex. However, other studies have reported no differences in NAA, Cho or Cr levels between patients and controls [59,60]. Bartha et al. conducted ^1H spectroscopy of the frontal lobes in drug-naive schizophrenics [61]. Compared with controls, the patients had increased levels of glutamine, although no differences in the levels of NAA or other studied chemicals were observed. Conversely, Cecil et al. reported that drug-naive patients had reduced NAA/Cr levels in frontal regions, together with increased Cho/Cr ratios [62]. No differences in amino acid/Cr ratios were observed between patients and controls, contradicting the findings of Bartha et al.

Taken together, these proton and phosphorus spectroscopy studies provide strong evidence for aberrant neuronal structure and function in schizophrenia, consistent with findings from other imaging modalities of structural [34] and functional [36] abnormalities.

Spectroscopy of the temporal lobes

As with structural imaging studies, MRS research has indicated abnormalities in temporal lobe neurochemistry. In a similar vein to studies of the frontal lobes, ^{31}P spectroscopy studies have reported evidence of abnormal levels of various compounds. For example, in a study of drug-naive schizophrenics, Fukuzako et al. found higher levels of PDEs and lower levels of PMEs, together with increased PCr, but only in the left temporal lobe [63]. Evidence of changes in energy-related chemicals is contradictory: while some studies have reported reduced levels of ATP in the left temporal lobe [64]; others have found increased levels [65].

Maier et al. [66] performed proton spectroscopy of the anterior hippocampus, and reported reduced levels of NAA, Cr and Cho. Other studies, such as those by Bertolino et al. [57,67], have reported reduced NAA levels without altered Cr or Cho levels. Again, Cecil et al. reported reduced NAA levels in temporal lobe regions of drug-naive patients, together with increased amino acid/Cr ratios, indicating possible neurotransmitter abnormalities [62].

If NAA is a measure of neuronal integrity, then reduced NAA levels would be consistent with the volume reductions of temporal lobe structures identified in structural imaging. However, there is evidence that the story is more complicated than that. Deicken et al. reported evidence of bilaterally reduced NAA in a sample of schizophrenics [68]. However, in their sample, no significant differences in hippocampal volume were observed between patients and controls. A similar pattern has been observed in other studies [56,57]. These findings suggest that reduced levels of NAA do not simply reflect the effect of atrophy, but instead reflect a more subtle underlying change, such as the level of neuronal function.

Spectroscopy – medication and symptomatology

In this chapter and the preceding one, we have discussed evidence showing medication effects on both brain structure and vascular activity. One effect of antipsychotic drugs may be to alter levels of certain metabolites, and so MRS studies are beginning to investigate drug-induced changes in cerebral biochemistry, and how these findings may relate to clinical presentation.

In view of the known different effects of antipsychotic drugs on the size of the basal ganglia, and possibly also on the size of the thalamus, Heimberg et al. used proton spectroscopy to study frontal and temporal regions, the basal ganglia and thalamus, in schizophrenic patients administered different antipsychotic drugs [69]. Overall, no difference in frontal lobe, temporal lobe or basal ganglia NAA/Cr levels was observed in the schizophrenics. However, a slight reduction in NAA/Cr in the thalamus was found, consistent with reports of reduced thalamic volume [70]. In relation to treatment effects, higher NAA levels were found in the left prefrontal cortex of patients on atypical drugs, compared with those on typical medication. It may be that atypical drugs are less neurotoxic than typical ones [71] and therefore might result in higher NAA levels. Volz et al. found that those on typical neuroleptics had increased levels of chemicals associated with energy usage compared with drug-free patients [32]. High levels of these metabolites were also linked to negative symptoms. This ties in with studies that have found hypofrontality to be associated with negative symptomatology [13].

In a recent study, Fukuzako et al. conducted a follow-up study of drug-naive patients in order to assess the effects of short-term antipsychotic treatment [72]. Using phosphorus spectroscopy of the temporal lobes, they showed that increased levels of phosphodiesters in patients were reduced following treatment with haloperidol, although still remaining above the levels seen in controls. This reduction was associated with a reduction in psychotic symptoms.

As with so many aspects of brain imaging in schizophrenia, MRS studies regularly produce conflicting results. Therefore, studies have begun to look at subgroups in the hope of identifying more consistent and neurobiologically relevant results. Shiori et al. performed ^{31}P spectroscopy of the frontal lobes in different subgroups of schizophrenics, and showed that reduced frontal lobe PME and increased PDE levels were linked to motor poverty, emotional withdrawal and blunted affect [73], consistent with structural and functional imaging studies that have linked frontal lobe dysfunction with negative symptoms. Similarly, in a proton spectroscopy study, Fukuzako et al. showed that patients diagnosed with a disorganised syndrome exhibited pronounced biochemical changes in the left medial temporal lobe compared with patients with a diagnosis of paranoid schizophrenia [74].

Spectroscopy – relationship to cognitive function
As with symptomatology, it is unclear the extent to which cognitive function may be linked to levels of particular chemicals. Using ^{31}P spectroscopy, Deicken et al. found that performance on the WCST was linked to frontal lobe PME levels in schizophrenics — lower frontal lobe PME levels were associated with poorer performance in terms of errors and category completion [75]. In contrast, again using ^{31}P spectroscopy, Volz et al. found no correlation between PME or PDE levels and WCST performance [76]. However, in controls, levels of PCr were negatively correlated with scores on the WCST. High levels of PCr are linked to reduced energy usage, so reduced usage was therefore linked to poorer performance.

A recent study investigated whether levels of brain chemicals were linked to other measures of brain function. There is evidence of abnormal working memory in schizophrenia and that this is characterised by hypofrontality in the dorsolateral prefrontal cortex [27,29,33,47]. Additionally, MRS studies have identified biochemical changes in this region, such as reduced levels of NAA [57,58]. Bertolino et al. investigated whether there was a relationship between proton spectroscopy measurements of the dorsolateral prefrontal cortex and working memory function [77]. They obtained PET scans of schizophrenics while performing two working memory tasks. The results showed that the NAA/Cr ratio in the prefrontal cortex was strongly and selectively correlated with brain activity in the prefrontal and parietal cortices (regions known to be involved in working memory) during the working memory tasks. No other spectroscopy signals were associated with activity in a working memory network. In addition, MRS measures in other regions — including areas involved in working memory — were not correlated with activity in any part of the network. These results show that the structural integrity of one region is related to distributed brain function, and provide further evidence to support abnormal neural circuits involving the prefrontal cortex.

Conclusions

PET and SPECT allow us to visualize occupancy of receptors by antipsychotic drugs in vivo, and to investigate how this relates to side-effects and symptomatology. Using these neuroimaging techniques it has been shown that high levels of D_2 receptor antagonism are linked to a high incidence of side effects, but not to clinical efficacy. Based on results from PET and SPECT studies, it has been suggested that a higher level of 5-HT$_2$ receptor occupancy by atypical medications may explain the improved side-effect profile of these drugs and their benefits on cognition, although high levels of 5-HT$_2$ blockade are not associated with clinical response. PET, SPECT and fMRI can be used to examine abnormal brain activity during cognitive tasks and during active and remitted psychosis, and to visualize the effects of antipsychotic drugs. Functional imaging studies suggest that there is abnormal connectivity in schizophrenia. MRS studies have shown abnormalities in neurotransmitter systems, neuronal membrane constituents and chemicals linked to energy metabolism. Future brain imaging work should further elucidate the links between brain function, cognitive function, symptomatology and medication.

References

1. Carlsson A. Antipsychotic drugs, neurotransmitters, and schizophrenia. *Am J Psychiatry* 1978;**135**:165–73.
2. Farde L, Wiesel FA, Halldin C et al. Central D_2-dopamine receptor occupancy in schizophrenic patients treated with antipsychotic drugs. *Arch Gen Psychiatry* 1988;**45**:71–6.
3. Bigliani V, Mulligan RS, Acton PD et al. In vivo occupancy of striatal and temporal cortical D2/D3 dopamine receptors by typical antipsychotic drugs. [123I]epidepride single photon emission tomography (SPET) study. *Br J Psychiatry* 1999;**175**:231–8.
4. Kapur S, Zipursky R, Jones C et al. Relationship between dopamine D(2) occupancy, clinical response, and side effects: a double-blind PET study of first-episode schizophrenia. *Am J Psychiatry* 2000;**157**:514–20.
5. Kapur S, Zipursky RB, Remington G. Clinical and theoretical implications of 5-HT$_2$ and D_2 receptor occupancy of clozapine, risperidone, and olanzapine in schizophrenia. *Am J Psychiatry* 1999;**156**:286–93.
6. Broich K, Grunwald F, Kasper S et al. D_2-dopamine receptor occupancy measured by IBZM-SPECT in relation to extrapyramidal side effects. *Pharmacopsychiatry* 1998;**31**:159–62.
7. Kasper S, Tauscher J, Kufferle B et al. Sertindole and dopamine D_2 receptor occupancy in comparison to risperidone, clozapine and haloperidol—a ¹²³I-IBZM SPECT study. *Psychopharmacology* 1998;**136**:367–73.
8. Travis MJ, Busatto GF, Pilowsky LS et al. 5-HT$_{2A}$ receptor blockade in patients with schizophrenia treated with risperidone or clozapine. A SPET study using the novel 5-HT$_{2A}$ ligand ¹²³I-5-I-R-91150. *Br J Psychiatry* 1998;**173**:236–41.
9. Kapur S, Zipursky RB, Remington G et al. 5-HT$_2$ and D_2 receptor occupancy of olanzapine in schizophrenia: a PET investigation. *Am J Psychiatry* 1998;**155**:921–8.

10. Kapur S, Remington G, Zipursky RB et al. The D_2 dopamine receptor occupancy of risperidone and its relationship to extrapyramidal symptoms: a PET study. *Life Sci* 1995;**57**:PL103–7.

11. Nyberg S, Eriksson B, Oxenstierna G et al. Suggested minimal effective dose of risperidone based on PET-measured D_2 and $5\text{-}HT_{2A}$ receptor occupancy in schizophrenic patients. *Am J Psychiatry* 1999;**156**(6):869–75.

12. Liddle PF, Friston KJ, Frith CD et al. Patterns of cerebral blood flow in schizophrenia. *Br J Psychiatry* 1992;**160**:179–86.

13. Wolkin A, Sanfilipo M, Wolf AP et al. Negative symptoms and hypofrontality in chronic schizophrenia. *Arch Gen Psychiatry* 1992;**49**(12):959–65.

14. Schroder J, Buchsbaum MS, Siegel BV et al. Cerebral metabolic activity correlates of subsyndromes in chronic schizophrenia. *Schizophr Res* 1996;**19**:41–53.

15. McGuire PK, Shah GM, Murray RM. Increased blood flow in Broca's area during auditory hallucinations in schizophrenia. *Lancet* 1993;**342**:703–6.

16. Sabri O, Erkwoh R, Schreckenberger M et al. Correlation of positive symptoms exclusively to hyperperfusion or hypoperfusion of cerebral cortex in never-treated schizophrenics. *Lancet* 1997;**349**:1735–9.

17. Frith CD, Done DJ. Towards a neuropsychology of schizophrenia. *Br J Psychiatry* 1988;**153**:437–43.

18. McGuire PK, Silbersweig DA, Frith CD. Functional neuroanatomy of verbal self-monitoring. *Brain* 1996;**119**:907–17.

19. McGuire PK, Quested DJ, Spence SA et al. Pathophysiology of 'positive' thought disorder in schizophrenia. *Br J Psychiatry* 1998;**173**:231–5.20.

20. Woodruff PW, Wright IC, Shuriquie N et al. Structural brain abnormalities in male schizophrenics reflect fronto-temporal dissociation. *Psychol Med* 1997;**27**:1257–66.

21. Shenton ME, Kikinis R, Jolesz FA et al. Abnormalities of the left temporal lobe and thought disorder in schizophrenia. A quantitative magnetic resonance imaging study. *New Engl J Med* 1992;**327**:604–12.

22. Dierks T, Linden DE, Jandl M et al. Activation of Heschl's gyrus during auditory hallucinations. *Neuron* 1999;**22**(3):615-21.

23. Spence SA, Hirsch SR, Brooks DJ et al. Prefrontal cortex activity in people with schizophrenia and control subjects. Evidence from positron emission tomography for remission of 'hypofrontality' with recovery from acute schizophrenia. *Br J Psychiatry* 1998;**172**:316–23.

24. Erkwoh R, Sabri O, Willmes K et al. Active and remitted schizophrenia: psychopathological and regional cerebral blood flow findings. *Psychiatry Res (Neuroimaging)* 1999;**90**:17–30.

25. Ingvar DH, Franzen G. Distribution of cerebral activity in chronic schizophrenia. *Lancet* 1974; **2**(7895):1484-6.

26. Andreasen NC, O'Leary DS, Flaum M et al. Hypofrontality in schizophrenia: distributed dysfunctional circuits in neuroleptic-naive patients. *Lancet* 1997;**349**(9067):1730–4.

27. Andreasen NC, Rezai K, Alliger R et al. Hypofrontality in neuroleptic-naive patients and in patients with chronic schizophrenia. Assessment with xenon 133 single-photon emission computed tomography and the Tower of London. *Arch Gen Psychiatry* 1992;**49**(12):943–58.

28. Carter CS, Perlstein W, Ganguli R et al. Functional hypofrontality and working memory dysfunction in schizophrenia. *Am J Psychiatry* 1998;**155**:1285–7.

29. Weinberger DR, Berman KF, Zec RF. Physiologic dysfunction of dorsolateral prefrontal cortex in schizophrenia. I. Regional cerebral blood flow evidence. *Arch Gen Psychiatry* 1986;**43**(2):114–24.

30. Heckers S, Rauch SL, Goff D et al. Impaired recruitment of the hippocampus during conscious recollection in schizophrenia. *Nat Neurosci* 1998;**1**(4):318–23.

31. Heckers S, Goff D, Schacter DL et al. Functional imaging of memory retrieval in deficit vs nondeficit schizophrenia. *Arch Gen Psychiatry* 1999;**56**(12):1117–23.

32. Volz HP, Gaser C, Hager F et al. Brain activation during cognitive stimulation with the Wisconsin Card Sorting Test—a functional MRI study on healthy volunteers and schizophrenics. *Psychiatry Res* 1997;**75**:145–57.

33. Stevens AA, Goldman-Rakic PS, Gore JC et al. Cortical dysfunction in schizophrenia during auditory word and tone working memory demonstrated by functional magnetic resonance imaging. *Arch Gen Psychiatry* 1998;**55**:1097–103.

34. Buchanan RW, Vladar K, Barta PE et al. Structural evaluation of the prefrontal cortex in schizophrenia. *Am J Psychiatry* 1998;**155**:1049–55.

35. Yurgelun-Todd DA, Waternaux CM et al. Functional magnetic resonance imaging of schizophrenic patients and comparison subjects during word production. *Am J Psychiatry* 1996;**153**:200–5.

36. Curtis VA, Bullmore ET, Brammer MJ et al. Attenuated frontal activation during a verbal fluency task in patients with schizophrenia. *Am J Psychiatry* 1998;**155**:1056–63.

37. Curtis VA, Bullmore ET, Morris RG et al. Attenuated frontal activation in schizophrenia may be task dependent. *Schizophr Res* 1999;**37**:35–44.

38. Wiser AK, Andreasen NC, O'Leary DS et al. Dysfunctional cortico-cerebellar circuits cause 'cognitive dysmetria' in schizophrenia. *Neuroreport* 1998;**9**:1895–99.

39. Andreasen NC, Paradiso S, O'Leary DS. "Cognitive dysmetria" as an integrative theory of schizophrenia: a dysfunction in cortical-subcortical-cerebellar circuitry? *Schizophr Bull* 1998;**24**:203–18.

40. Jennings JM, McIntosh AR, Kapur S et al. Functional network differences in schizophrenia: a rCBF study of semantic processing. *Neuroreport* 1998;**9**:1697–700.

41. Fletcher P, McKenna PJ, Friston KJ et al. Abnormal cingulate modulation of fronto-temporal connectivity in schizophrenia. *Neuroimage* 1999; **9**(3):337-42.

42. Spence SA, Liddle PF, Stefan MD et al. Functional anatomy of verbal fluency in people with schizophrenia and those at genetic risk. Focal dysfunction and distributed disconnectivity reappraised. *Br J Psychiatry* 2000;**176**:52–60.

43. Buchsbaum MS, Tang CY, Peled S et al. MRI white matter diffusion anisotropy and PET metabolic rate in schizophrenia. *Neuroreport* 1998;**9**(3):425–30.

44. Buchsbaum MS, Hazlett EA, Haznedar MM et al. Visualizing fronto-striatal circuitry and neuroleptic effects in schizophrenia. *Acta Psychiatr Scand Suppl* 1999;**395**:129–37.

45. Chakos MH, Lieberman JA, Bilder RM et al. Increase in caudate nuclei volumes of first-episode schizophrenic patients taking antipsychotic drugs. *Am J Psychiatry* 1994;**151**:1430–6.

46. Miller DD, Andreasen NC, O'Leary DS et al. Effect of antipsychotics on regional cerebral blood flow measured with positron emission tomography. *Neuropsychopharmacology* 1997;**17**:230–40.

47. Honey GD, Bullmore ET, Soni W et al. Differences in frontal cortical activation by a working memory task after substitution of risperidone for typical antipsychotic drugs in patients with schizophrenia. *Proc Natl Acad Sci USA* 1999;**96**(23):13432–7.

48. Watanabe M, Kodama T, Hikosaka K. Increase of extracellular dopamine in primate prefrontal cortex during a working memory task. *J Neurophysiol* 1997;**78**(5):2795–8.

49. Hertel P, Nomikos GG, Iurlo M et al. Risperidone: regional effects in vivo on release and metabolism of dopamine and serotonin in the rat brain. *Psychopharmacology (Berl)* 1996;**124**(152):74–86.

50. Meltzer HY, McGurk SR. The effects of clozapine, risperidone, and olanzapine on cognitive function in schizophrenia. *Schizophr Bull* 1999;**25**(2):233–55.

51. Kegeles LS, Humaran TJ, Mann JJ. In vivo neurochemistry of the brain in schizophrenia as revealed by magnetic resonance spectroscopy. *Biol Psychiatry* 1998;**44**:382–98.

52. Pettegrew JW, Keshavan MS, Panchalingam K et al. Alterations in brain high-energy phosphate and membrane phospholipid metabolism in first-episode, drug-naive schizophrenics. A pilot study of the dorsal prefrontal cortex by in vivo phosphorus 31 nuclear magnetic resonance spectroscopy. *Arch Gen Psychiatry* 1991;**48**:563–8.

53. Williamson P, Drost D, Stanley J et al. Localized phosphorous 31 magnetic resonance spectroscopy in chronic schizophrenic patients and normal controls. *Arch Gen Psychiatry* 1991;**48**(6):578.

54. Deicken RF, Calabrese G, Merrin EL et al. 31 phosphorus magnetic resonance spectroscopy of the frontal and parietal lobes in chronic schizophrenia. *Biol Psychiatry* 1994;**36**:503–10.

55. Potwarka JJ, Drost DJ, Williamson PC et al. A 1H-decoupled 31P chemical shift imaging study of medicated schizophrenic patients and healthy controls. *Biol Psychiatry* 1999; **45**(6):687-93

56. Deicken RF, Zhou L, Corwin F et al. Decreased left frontal lobe N-acetylaspartate in schizophrenia. *Am J Psychiatry* 1997;**154**:688–90.

57. Bertolino A, Nawroz S, Mattay VS et al. Regionally specific pattern of neurochemical pathology in schizophrenia as assessed by multislice proton magnetic resonance spectroscopic imaging. *Am J Psychiatry* 1996;**153**:1554–63.

58. Bertolino A, Callicott JH, Elman I et al. Regionally specific neuronal pathology in untreated patients with schizophrenia: a proton magnetic resonance spectroscopic imaging study. *Biol Psychiatry* 1998;**43**:641–8.

59. Buckley PF, Moore C, Long H et al. ^{1}H-magnetic resonance spectroscopy of the left temporal and frontal lobes in schizophrenia: clinical, neurodevelopmental, and cognitive correlates. *Biol Psychiatry* 1994;**36**:792–800.

60. Fukuzako H, Takeuchi K, Hokazono Y et al. Proton magnetic resonance spectroscopy of the left medial temporal and frontal lobes in chronic schizophrenia: preliminary report. *Psychiatry Res (Neuroimaging)* 1995;**61**:193–200.

61. Bartha R, Williamson PC, Drost DJ et al. Measurement of glutamate and glutamine in the medial prefrontal cortex of never-treated schizophrenic patients and healthy controls by proton magnetic resonance spectroscopy. *Arch Gen Psychiatry* 1997;**54**:959–65.

62. Cecil KM, Lenkinski RE, Gur RE, Gur RC. Proton magnetic resonance spectroscopy in the frontal and temporal lobes of neuroleptic naive patients with schizophrenia. *Neuropsychopharmacology* 1999;**20**:131–40.

63. Fukuzako H, Fukuzako T, Hashiguchi T et al. Changes in levels of phosphorus metabolites in temporal lobes of drug-naive schizophrenic patients. *Am J Psychiatry* 1999;**156**(8):1205–8.

64. Fukuzako H, Takeuchi K, Ueyama K et al. ^{31}P magnetic resonance spectroscopy of the medial temporal lobe of schizophrenic patients with neuroleptic-resistant marked positive symptoms. *Eur Arch Psychiatry Clin Neurosci* 1994;**244**(5):236–40.

65. Deicken RF, Calabrese G, Merrin EL et al. Asymmetry of temporal lobe phosphorous metabolism in schizophrenia: a 31 phosphorous magnetic resonance spectroscopic imaging study. *Biol Psychiatry* 1995;**38**(5):279–86.

66. Maier M, Ron MA, Barker GJ et al. Proton magnetic resonance spectroscopy: an in vivo method of estimating hippocampal neuronal depletion in schizophrenia. *Psychol Med* 1995;**25**:1201–9.

67. Mattay VS, Callicott JH, Bertolino A et al. Abnormal functional lateralization of the sensorimotor cortex in patients with schizophrenia. *Neuroreport* 1997;**8**:2977–84.

68. Deicken RF, Pegues M, Amend D. Reduced hippocampal N-acetylaspartate without volume loss in schizophrenia. *Schizophr Res* 1999;**37**(3):217–23.

69. Heimberg C, Komoroski RA, Lawson WB et al. Regional proton magnetic resonance spectroscopy in schizophrenia and exploration of drug effect. *Psychiatry Res (Neuroimaging)* 1998;**83**:105–15.

70. Andreasen NC, Arndt S, Swayze V et al. Thalamic abnormalities in schizophrenia visualized through magnetic resonance image averaging. *Science* 1994;**266**:294–8.

71. Fujimura M, Hashimoto K, Yamagami K. Effects of antipsychotic drugs on neurotoxicity, expression of fos-like protein and c-fos mRNA in the retrosplenial cortex after administration of dizocilpine. *Eur J Pharmacol* 2000;**398**(1):1-10.

72. Fukuzako H, Fukuzako T, Kodama S et al. Haloperidol improves membrane phospholipid abnormalities in temporal lobes of schizophrenic patients. *Neuropsychopharmacology* 1999;**21**(4):542–9.

73. Shioiri T, Someya T, Murashita J et al. Multiple regression analysis of relationship between frontal lobe phsophorus metabolism and clinical symptoms in patients with schizophrenia. *Psychiatry Res* 1997;**76**(2–3):113–22.

74. Fukuzako H, Kodama S, Fukuzako T et al. Subtype-associated metabolite differences in the temporal lobe in schizophrenia detected by proton magnetic resonance spectroscopy. *Psychiatry Res* 1999;**92**(1):45–56.

75. Deicken RF, Calabrese G, Merrin EL et al. Asymmetry of temporal lobe phosphorous metabolism in schizophrenia: a 31 phosphorous magnetic resonance spectroscopic imaging study. *Biol Psychiatry* 1995;**38**(5):279–86.

76. Volz HP, Hubner G, Rzanny R et al. High-energy phosphates in the frontal lobe correlate with Wisconsin Card Sort Test performance in controls, not in schizophrenics: a 31 phosphorus magnetic resonance spectroscopic and neuropsychological investigation. *Schizophr Res* 1998;**31**:37–47.

77. Bertolino A, Esposito G, Callicott JH et al. Specific relationship between prefrontal neuronal N-acetylaspartate and activation of the working memory cortical network in schizophrenia. *Am J Psychiatry* 2000;**157**(1):26–33.

CHAPTER 5
Genetics and Brain Imaging in Schizophrenia

Genetics of schizophrenia

To what extent is susceptibility to schizophrenia genetically influenced? It is clear that closeness, in genetic terms, to an affected individual increases a person's chances of developing the illness. Figures such as a prevalence of 1% in the adult population, 8–10% in siblings of patients, and 12–15% in children of patients lend support to the idea of a genetic component in the aetiology of schizophrenia. However, identical twins only show a 50% concordance rate, rather than the 100% that would be expected in an entirely genetically transmitted disorder, showing that non-genetic factors must play an important part. It is unclear whether genetic factors predispose individuals to schizophrenia directly, or rather to an increased cerebral sensitivity to noxious events such as hypoxia, infection and febrile seizures. Lesions thus produced might eventually manifest themselves as schizophrenia. Brain imaging studies have been used to study various familial relationships in schizophrenia, in the hope of identifying genetic risk factors for the illness; i.e. structural or functional abnormalities in patients and their relatives that may be genetically transmitted.

Twin studies

30% of our genes are expressed solely in the brain, and so it is hardly surprising to find out that genes play a very important role in controlling the development of the brain. Principally this evidence has come from studies of monozygotic and dizygotic twins. Cerebral volume has been shown to be extremely highly genetically determined [1] and there is also evidence for significant genetic influences on regional cortical and subcortical volumes [2]. Other studies have begun to investigate the degree to which patterns of cortical folding may be determined by genes. Thus far there is evidence for a high degree of similarity of sulcal patterns within identical twin pairs, suggesting that these are also under predominantly genetic control [3,4]. Given that identical twins possess exactly the same genes — although Tsujita et al. suggest that this is not entirely true [5] — studies of discordant twin pairs, i.e. where one twin is schizophrenic and the other is not, provide a fascinating insight into the links between genetic and environmental contributions and disease state. Given that identical twins may have completely separate chorions or amnions (the membranous sacs enclosing the foetus), there are a number of factors that might account for discordance among identical twins e.g.:

• Chromosome or gene changes occurring after cleavage of the zygote
• Differences in blood circulation and oxygenation occurring during gestation and at birth, leading to differential exposure to infectious agents, drugs or chemicals during gestation

Indeed, it appears that concordant monozygotic twins (i.e. where both are schizophrenic) are more likely to have been monochorionic and to have shared a

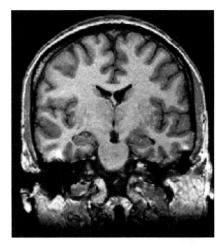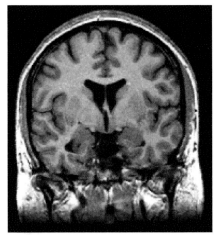

Figure 1. Magnetic resonance imaging (MRI) scan of a well twin (left) and his schizophrenic twin (right). Structural brain abnormalities associated with schizophrenia are clearly shown on these MRI images. The schizophrenic individual has enlarged ventricles and cortical sulci.

single placenta during gestation. Thus, sharing the same foetal blood circulation would offer equal exposure to pre-birth infections, a factor that would be consistent with the hypothesis of foetal viral infection in the aetiology of schizophrenia [6].

A number of studies have used different brain imaging techniques to contrast brain structure and function in twins discordant for schizophrenia. These studies support the notion that development of schizophrenia is partly, but only partly, genetically determined. In terms of brain structure, there is evidence that the affected twin in a discordant pair exhibits more severe structural abnormalities, such as increased ventricular size [7] and reduced cerebral [8] and hippocampal volume [9], than the unaffected twin (Figure 1).

In terms of brain function, a positron emission tomography (PET) study of regional cerebral blood flow (rCBF) during performance of the Wisconsin Card Sorting Test found that affected twins exhibited hypofrontality (reduced activity of prefrontal regions) whereas their unaffected twins did not — the unaffected siblings being indistinguishable from control twins [10]. In a similar vein, neuropsychological assessment of twins discordant for the disorder revealed that, in many domains of function, the affected twin showed significantly more impairment than the well twin, although some differences between well twins and healthy controls were observed [11]. All of this suggests that structural and functional abnormalities may be partially genetically mediated, and that there must be a secondary process, acting in addition to genetic factors, that leads to the development of psychosis.

Family studies
Studies of families with multiple generations affected by schizophrenia offer a unique insight into the pathogenesis of the disorder. In these families it is often possible to identify a *presumed obligate carrier*, someone who is assumed to carry the schizophrenia gene(s) but is not affected with the illness. Structural and

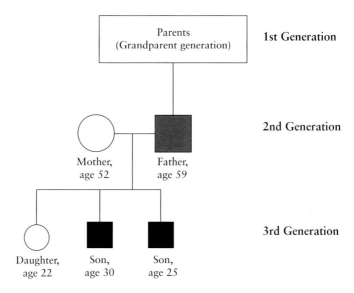

Figure 2. A typical inheritance pattern of a family multiply affected with schizophrenia. Here, males are represented by squares and females by circles. The male represented by the red square is a parent of the third generation and is the presumed obligate carrier. He suffers from a schizotypal personality disorder and comes from a lineage in which one of his parents and/or family members suffered from psychiatric illness/es. His wife does not have a family history of psychiatric illness. Amongst their children, two sons have been diagnosed as schizophrenic whilst the daughter is unaffected.

functional imaging studies of relatives, such as presumed obligate carriers and siblings of schizophrenics, may help to identify biological markers for the illness. Sharma et al. [12–14] carried out a series of studies of brain abnormalities in families multiply affected with schizophrenia. A typical family pattern from the study is shown in Figure 2.

The authors hypothesized that:

1. Schizophrenic probands would exhibit more structural brain abnormalities than normal controls
2. Presumed obligate carriers would show similar abnormalities to the schizophrenics
3. Unaffected offspring of schizophrenic parent/s would also exhibit structural abnormalities
4. Schizophrenics would exhibit more extensive structural brain abnormalities than their siblings

The structural brain images (MRI) shown in Figures 3–6 clearly illustrate these points.

There is evidence that schizophrenics, presumed obligate carriers and unaffected siblings manifest some of the structural abnormalities associated with schizophrenia, although abnormalities may be more frequent in schizophrenics than in first-degree relatives and controls (Figure 7) [12]. In particular, presumed obligate

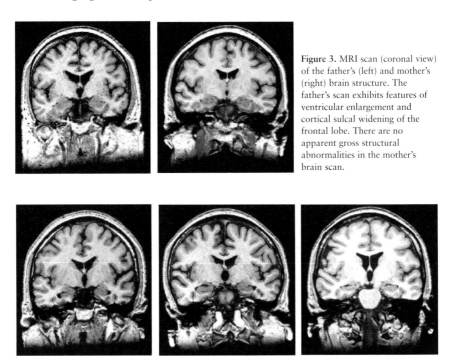

Figure 3. MRI scan (coronal view) of the father's (left) and mother's (right) brain structure. The father's scan exhibits features of ventricular enlargement and cortical sulcal widening of the frontal lobe. There are no apparent gross structural abnormalities in the mother's brain scan.

Figure 4. MRI scan (coronal view) of the three offspring — oldest son, youngest son and daughter (left to right). Both sons exhibit the classic findings of structural brain abnormalities — ventricular enlargement and asymmetry and widening of the interhemispheric fissure and sulcal spaces. The daughter's scan also exhibits enlarged ventricles, the brain anatomy appearing otherwise relatively normal.

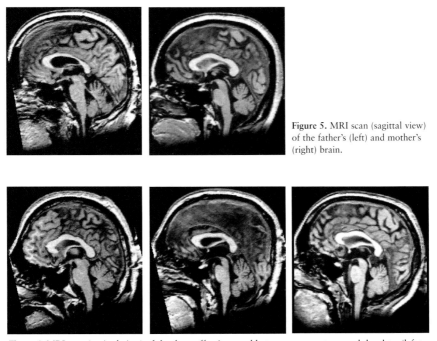

Figure 5. MRI scan (sagittal view) of the father's (left) and mother's (right) brain.

Figure 6. MRI scan (sagittal view) of the three offspring — oldest son, youngest son and daughter (left to right).

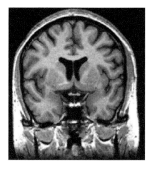 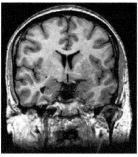

Figure 7. Coronal view of a schizophrenic male (left) and his unaffected sibling (right). Again, the brain of the affected sibling shows ventricular and sulcal enlargement.

carriers appear to have increased lateral ventricular volume, which may reflect a genetic predisposition to schizophrenia — a schizophrenia endophenotype [13]. There is also evidence that normal cerebral asymmetries, which have been reported to be lost in schizophrenics [15], may also be missing in their relatives, suggesting that the genes that control their patterning may be abnormally expressed in schizophrenia [14]. Other studies have reported reduced cortical grey matter volumes and increased sulcal cerebrospinal fluid volumes [16], increased third ventricular volume [17], reduced thalamic volume [18] and reduced hippocampal and amygdala volumes [19] in first-degree relatives compared with controls.

There is also evidence of functional abnormalities in first degree relatives of schizophrenics. A recent study used PET to investigate brain activity in schizophrenics and a group of presumed obligate carriers [20]. During a verbal fluency task, no significant differences in brain activity were observed between the obligate carriers and controls. However, when connections between brain regions were studied, obligate carriers were shown to have reduced connectivity between the left prefrontal cortex and precuneus. There were also qualitative differences between obligate carriers, patients and controls in terms of abnormal lateralisation of activation (discussed in Crow et al. [21]). Another study looked at the functional correlates of deficits in eye-movements in relatives of schizophrenics [22]. The study looked at two groups of relatives, those who showed deficits in smooth pursuit (the ability to follow a moving target, such as a light), and those who did not. Smooth pursuit deficits have been shown to be a fairly reliable marker of genetic risk for schizophrenia [23]. The results showed that relatives with deficient smooth pursuit showed markedly less activation of a prefrontal region (the frontal eye fields) than controls, or relatives with normal pursuit. This is interesting, as it identifies the underlying biological substrate of a possible genetic marker. Lastly, there is evidence from one spectroscopy study of chemical abnormalities in the brains of siblings, in the form of reduced N-acetyl aspartate (NAA) in the hippocampus, suggesting underlying neuronal dysfunction [24].

Studies of the offspring of schizophrenics, at high risk of developing schizophrenia, have also provided evidence for a genetic risk factor. These studies have identified structural abnormalities in the form of reduced amygdala and thalamic volumes [25], reduced cerebral volume and increased volume of the third ventricle, and functional abnormalities in the form of a reduced NAA/choline ratio in the anterior cingulate [26].

Together with the twin studies described earlier, it is clear that genetic susceptibility to schizophrenia is expressed in the form of structural and functional brain abnormalities, but that some additional non-genetic factors must be important in the transition to schizophrenia.

Genetic and non-genetic effects on brain structure

Because structural and functional abnormalities found in schizophrenics seem to be at least partially genetically mediated, studies are beginning to investigate links between genes and brain structure and function. This work stems from the study of disorders where the genetic abnormality is known, such as in Williams syndrome [27]. Although no abnormal genes have definitely been found for schizophrenia, a recent study has tried to link genes with structural abnormalities in schizophrenia [29]. This study examined a particular genetic pattern (a dinucleotide repeat) in a gene, NT-3 (neurotrophin-3), that is involved in cell proliferation and migration, and is particularly highly expressed in the hippocampus [29]. This polymorphism has been reported to be more common in schizophrenics than in controls [30]. The study showed that schizophrenics who carried the particular allele of the NT-3 gene had smaller hippocampal volumes than schizophrenics who did not.

However, it is also important to remember that other, non-genetic factors may play a significant role in producing the structural abnormalities associated with schizophrenia. Although the study described above [28], together with twin [9] and family studies [31], suggests that abnormalities in the hippocampus may be genetically mediated, a recent study has suggested that the story may be more complicated [30]. This study examined the volume of the hippocampus in two groups of schizophrenics: one group from multiply affected families (i.e. a group where genetic factors are likely to predominate), and another group with no familial history of schizophrenia, but with a history of obstetric complications. The results showed that only schizophrenics with a history of obstetric complications had reduced hippocampal volume compared with controls. There is also evidence for this from a study of twins discordant for schizophrenia, which showed that labour complications were associated with structural abnormalities such as larger ventricles and smaller hippocampal volumes [33]. This suggests that hippocampal abnormalities may not only reflect a genetic cause, and shows how difficult it is to dissect the contributions of genetic and environmental factors in the aetiology of schizophrenia.

Complexity of schizophrenia genetics

Recognition of a strong genetic influence in schizophrenia raises questions regarding the nature of this influence (reviewed in DeLisi et al. [34]). Research has established that schizophrenia does not follow classic Mendelian inheritance. The disorder exhibits reduced penetrance: despite a high genetic liability, disease manifestation may not occur. Contrary to Mendelian inheritance, schizophrenic phenocopies exist, i.e. instances in which schizophrenic-like symptoms are produced by metabolic or neurological conditions or drug abuse.

It is clear that schizophrenia is a highly complex and heterogeneous disorder, with defects at many genes possibly involved in producing the spectrum of schizophrenic illnesses. It is also clear from the twin and family studies described above that genes that influence susceptibility to schizophrenia exist in the human genome. However, their number and magnitude of effect remain to be determined. Brain imaging techniques have a major role to play in understanding what structural and functional changes are genetically transmitted. Currently we know that relatives show some of the structural and functional changes seen in schizophrenics. However, much remains unclear. It may eventually be possible to identify reliable risk markers for the disorder. Additionally, there is already evidence that genetic make-up may be linked to antipsychotic drug response [36]. As structural and functional imaging become increasingly used in planning and monitoring pharmacotherapy, integrating imaging studies with genetic research should help to elucidate the relationship between genes and cerebral structure and function. Research into these areas will have both theoretical and clinical significance.

References

1. Bartley AJ, Jones DW, Weinberger DR. Genetic variability of human brain size and cortical gyral patterns. *Brain* 1997;**120**(Pt 2):257-69.
2. Pennington BF, Filipek PA, Lefly D et al. A twin study of size variations in human brain. *J Cogn Neurosci* 2000;**12**(1):223-32.
3. Lohmann G, von Cramon DY, Steinmetz H. Sulcal variability of twins. *Cereb Cortex* 1999;**9**(7):754-63.
4. Le Goualher G, Argenti AM, Duyme M et al. Statistical sulcal shape comparisons: application to the detection of genetic encoding of the central sulcus shape. *Neuroimage* 2000;**11**(5 Pt 1):564-74.
5. Tsujita T, Niikawa N, Yamashita H et al. Genomic discordance between monozygotic twins discordant for schizophrenia. *Am J Psychiatry* 1998;**155**:422–4.
6. Davis JO, Phelps JA. Twins with schizophrenia: genes or germs? *Schizophr Bull* 1995;**21**:13–8.
7. Ohara K, Xu HD, Matsunaga T et al. Cerebral ventricle-brain ratio in monozygotic twins discordant and concordant for schizophrenia. *Prog Neuropsychopharmacol Biol Psychiatry* 1998;**22**:1043–50.
8. Noga JT, Bartley AJ, Jones DW et al. Cortical gyral anatomy and gross brain dimensions in monozygotic twins discordant for schizophrenia. *Schizophr Res* 1996;**22**:27–40.
9. Suddath RL, Christison GW, Torrey EF et al. Anatomical abnormalities in the brains of monozygotic twins discordant for schizophrenia. *New Engl J Med* 1990;**322**:789–94.
10. Berman KF, Torrey EF, Daniel DG et al. Regional cerebral blood flow in monozygotic twins discordant and concordant for schizophrenia. *Arch Gen Psychiatry* 1992;**49**:927–34.
11. Goldberg TE, Ragland JD, Torrey EF et al. Neuropsychological assessment of monozygotic twins discordant for schizophrenia. *Arch Gen Psychiatry* 1990;**47**(11):1066–72.
12. Sharma T, DuBoulay G, Lewis S et al. The Maudsley Family Study. I: Structural brain changes on magnetic resonance imaging in familial schizophrenia. *Prog Neuropsychopharmacol Biol Psychiatry* 1997;**21**:1297–315.
13. Sharma T, Lancaster E, Lee D et al. Brain changes in schizophrenia. Volumetric MRI study of families multiply affected with schizophrenia—the Maudsley Family Study 5. *Br J Psychiatry* 1998;**173**:132–8.
14. Sharma T, Lancaster E, Sigmundsson T et al. Lack of normal pattern of cerebral asymmetry in familial schizophrenic patients and their relatives—The Maudsley Family Study. *Schizophr Res* 1999;**40**(2):111–20.
15. Bilder RM, Wu H, Bogerts B et al. Absence of regional hemispheric volume asymmetries in first-episode schizophrenia. *Am J Psychiatry* 1994;**151**:1437–47.
16. Cannon TD, van Erp TG, Huttunen M et al. Regional gray matter, white matter, and cerebrospinal fluid distributions in schizophrenic patients, their siblings, and controls. *Arch Gen Psychiatry* 1998;**55**:1084–91.

17. Staal WG, Pol HE, Schnack HG et al. Structural brain abnormalities in patients with schizophrenia and their healthy siblings. *Am J Psychiatry* 2000;**157**:416–21.

18. Staal WG, Hulshoff PH, Schnack H et al. Partial volume decrease of the thalamus in relatives of patients with schizophrenia. *Am J Psychiatry* 1998;**155**:1784–6.

19. Seidman LJ, Faraone SV, Goldstein JM et al. Thalamic and amygdala-hippocampal volume reductions in first-degree relatives of patients with schizophrenia: an MRI-based morphometric analysis. *Biol Psychiatry* 1999;**46**(7):941–54.

20. Spence SA, Liddle PF, Stefan MD et al. Functional anatomy of verbal fluency in people with schizophrenia and those at genetic risk. *Br J Psychiatry* 2000;**176**:52–60.

21. Crow TJ. Invited commentary on: Functional anatomy of verbal fluency in people with schizophrenia and those at genetic risk. *Br J Psychiatry* 2000;**176**:61–3.

22. O'Driscoll GA, Benkelfat C, Florencio PS et al. Neural correlates of eye tracking deficits in first-degree relatives of schizophrenic patients: a positron emission tomography study. *Arch Gen Psychiatry* 1999;**56**(12):1127–34.

23. Keefe RS, Silverman JM, Mohs RC et al. Eye tracking, attention, and schizotypal symptoms in nonpsychotic relatives of patients with schizophrenia. *Arch Gen Psychiatry* 1997;**54**(2):169–76.

24. Callicott JH, Egan MF, Bertolino A et al. Hippocampal N-acetyl aspartate in unaffected siblings of patients with schizophrenia: a possible intermediate neurobiological phenotype. *Biol Psychiatry* 1998;**44**:941–50.

25. Lawrie SM, Whalley H, Kestelman JN, et al. Magnetic resonance imaging of brain in people at high risk of developing schizophrenia. *Lancet* 1999;**353**(9146):30–3.

26. Keshavan MS, Montrose DM, Pierri JN et al. Magnetic resonance imaging and spectroscopy in offspring at risk for schizophrenia: preliminary studies. *Prog Neuropsychopharmacol Biol Psychiatry* 1997;**21**:1285–95.

27. Bellugi U, Lichtenberger L, Mills D et al. Bridging cognition, the brain and molecular genetics: evidence from Williams syndrome. *Trends Neurosci* 1999;**2**(5):197–207.

28. Kunugi H, Hattori M, Nanko S et al. Dinucleotide repeat polymorphism in the neurotrophin-3 gene and hippocampal volume in psychoses. *Schizophr Res* 1999;**37**(3):271–3.

29. Maisonpierre PC, Belluscio L, Squinto S et al. Neurotrophin-3: a neurotrophic factor related to NGF and BDNF. *Science* 1990;**247**(4949 Pt 1):1446–51.

30. Jonsson E, Brene S, Zhang XR et al. Schizophrenia and neurotrophin-3 alleles. *Acta Psychiatr Scand* 1997;**95**(5):414–9.

31. Seidman LJ, Faraone SV, Goldstein JM et al. Reduced subcortical brain volumes in nonpsychotic siblings of schizophrenic patients: a pilot magnetic resonance imaging study. *Am J Med Genet* 1997;**74**(5):507–14.

32. Stefanis N, Frangou S, Yakeley J et al. Hippocampal volume reduction in schizophrenia: effects of genetic risk and pregnancy and birth complications. Biol *Psychiatry* 1999; **46**(5):697-702.

33. McNeil TF, Cantor-Graae E, Weinberger DR. Relationship of obstetric complications and differences in size of brain structures in monozygotic twin pairs discordant for schizophrenia. *Am J Psychiatry* 2000;**157**(2):203–12.

34. Tsuang M. Schizophrenia: genes and environment. *Biol Psychiatry* 2000;**47**(3):210-20.

35. Arranz MJ, Munro J, Sham P et al. Meta-analysis of studies on genetic variation in 5-HT$_{2A}$ receptors and clozapine response. *Schizophr Res* 1998;**32**(2):93–9.

Conclusion

Almost every aspect of research discussed in this book is littered with inconsistent findings. This is often passed off under the guise of the 'heterogeneity of schizophrenia', although this sheds little light on the illness itself. Nevertheless, imaging studies have provided important insight into the neurobiological correlates of this disease.

Structural magnetic resonance imaging (MRI) has identified the major regions that seem to be abnormal in schizophrenia. The development of analysis techniques such as high dimensional mapping, by allowing us to identify abnormal regions within a structure, will help us to characterize better the structural abnormalities present in psychiatric illness. Equally as important, structural imaging is beginning to unravel the presently poorly characterized links between medication, changes in brain structure and clinical efficacy. Thus far, drug effects have only been demonstrated on a few structures, although functional imaging studies have shown that drugs act much more diffusely. It may be that simple volumetric approaches are too crude to explore this sort of question; however, more sophisticated techniques may greatly advance our knowledge in this area. Attempts to correlate symptoms with brain structure have met with limited success — there is an obvious problem of linking a state phenomenon (symptoms) with a much more static one (brain structure). Studies of clinical subtypes may further elucidate this area, as, for example, functional imaging studies have shown that patients with a history of hallucinations may show different patterns of brain activation compared with those who have no such history. This is a very under-explored area in terms of structural imaging, and may help to explain some of the inconsistencies in the field.

Within the field of functional brain imaging, much current interest is being focused on functional MRI (fMRI) as a tool that will greatly enhance our understanding of normal brain functioning and how it may differ in psychiatric illnesses. While many researchers focus on exploring the cognitive deficits that often accompany schizophrenia, others are capitalizing on recent technical advances in order to image people when they are experiencing symptoms such as hallucinations. This sort of attempt to understand the state characteristics of schizophrenia may open new avenues in schizophrenia research. However, techniques such as positron emission tomography (PET) and single photon emission computed tomography (SPECT) still have a vital role to play. The ability to visualize neurotransmitter systems through receptor activity has greatly advanced our understanding of the new antipsychotic drugs. As neurochemical theories of schizophrenia have moved beyond a simple dopamine hypothesis, studies that concentrate on neurotransmitter-system interactions will play a major part in future research. Another growing area involves linking changes in brain function — either in terms of changes in receptor functioning or blood flow — with medication status, clinical improvement and cognitive functioning. Understanding the link between medication and brain function is vital to the development of the next generation of antipsychotic drugs.

Given the large number of brain structures that have been reported to be abnormal in schizophrenia, the focus of research has switched from lesion models of psychosis to theories of disordered neural circuitry. There is already evidence from both structural and functional studies of abnormal connections and interactions between brain regions in schizophrenia, which may help to explain the symptoms and cognitive deficits associated with this disease.

Magnetic resonance spectroscopy (MRS) has allowed us to take biochemistry away from post-mortem studies and to explore very small changes in molecular functioning in vivo in schizophrenia. With MRS we can directly study where drugs concentrate; this will provide clues about sites of pathology and about where new drugs should be targeted. We may also begin to identify predictors of treatment response and to map cognitive dysfunction onto localized neuronal dysfunction.

We know remarkably little about controlling influences on brain development. Although we know that many genes are expressed only in the brain, we know very little about how they may affect brain structure, both in normal people and in those with psychiatric disorders — imaging studies provide a unique opportunity to explore these and related questions. Advances in genetic research are providing great insights into the patterning processes involved in brain development. Studying how certain genetic patterns may affect brain structure should see imaging come together with genetics to help us understand better the origins of schizophrenia.

In terms of clinical practice, imaging has transformed our understanding of the mechanisms of action of antipsychotic medications, and therefore their clinical use. However, many questions remain to be answered. Why does a patient who has remained stable on medication for months, or possibly years, begin to develop symptoms again? What can predict relapse, and how can we best treat it? Why do some patients respond to one type of medication but not to another? Why are some patients unresponsive to any currently available neuroleptic? At the moment, we have very little understanding of the neurobiological correlates of relapse, remission and treatment response in schizophrenia. Neuroimaging offers us the possibility of answering these questions, and therefore improving the quality of patient care.

Index

adenosine diphosphate (ADP), neuronal activation 52

adenosine triphosphate (ATP), ^{31}P MRS assessment 22

alanine, chemical shift pattern 22

allergic reactions, radioligands
    PET contraindication 11
    SPECT contraindications 14

amino acids, MRS assessment 20-21

amygdala 28
    genetic influences 63
    MRI 7
    see also hippocampus—amygdala complex

amyotrophic lateral sclerosis (ALS), clinical management monitoring, MRS assessment 23

anaphylactic reactions, radioligands, PET contraindication 11

aneurysm clips
    MRI contraindication 5
    MRS contraindication 20

angiography, CT 4

anisotropy
    diffusion, MRI 8
    diffusion reduction, white matter changes 31

annihilation reaction, PET imaging 11

antidepressant medication, MRS assessment 23

antipsychotic medication
    5-HT$_2$ receptors 42-43
    basal ganglia 54-55
    brain region reactivation 51
    brain structure 29-30
        treatment response 30
    dopamine receptors
        antagonism 29
        blockade 41-44
    extrapyramidal side effects (EPS) 29, 41-42, 44
    MRS assessment 20, 23
    neuronal function influence 50-51
    neurotransmitter receptors 42
    PDE reduction 54
    rCBF 50
    short-term effects 54
    site of action
        PET imaging 11, 12
        SPECT imaging 14, 15
    STG volume reversal 30

aortic stents
    metallic, MRI contraindication 5
    MRS contraindication 20

aspartate, chemical shift pattern 22

axonal bundles
    anisotropy 8
    assessment, DWI 31
    myelination, MT 10

basal ganglia, antipsychotic medication, proton spectroscopy 54-55

blood-oxygenation-level-dependent (BOLD) effect, fMRI 17

brain function
    biochemistry, drug-induced changes 53-54
    energy processes, MRS assessment 20
    genetic influences 63
    NAA/choline ratio, anterior cingulate 63
    state 46-47
    twin studies 60, 64
    see also cerebral activity; cognitive function

brain imaging
    antipsychotic medication effect 50-52
    brain slice thickness, MRI 6-7
    and cognition
        fMRI 47-48
        PET and SPECT 11, 46-47
    functional 11-24, 41-58
    genetics of schizophrenia 59-66
    SPECT imaging 15-16
    structural 3-10, 25-40

brain mapping
    high-dimensional 32-36
    template brain 32
    variability map 32, 33

brain stem, MRI 7, 9

brain structure
    and antipsychotic medication 29-30, 51
    connectivity reduction, obligate carriers 63
    discordant twins 60
    dysconnectivity 30-31
    early disease 28
    fMRI mapping 18-19
    genetic and non-genetic effects 64
    surface CT imaging 4

brain tumours
    diagnosis
        MRS assessment 22
        PET imaging 11
    localization, fMRI 16-17

Broca's area, rCBF, auditory hallucinations 45

capsule, internal, MRI 9

carbon-13 (^{13}C) MRS 21, 23

caudate nucleus
    MRI 7, 9
    volume, neuroleptic therapy 29

cerebellum
    atrophy 25
    dysconnectivity 31
    MRI 7, 9

cerebral activity
    antipsychotic medication 50
    fMRI 45-46
        mapping 18-19
    PET and SPECT 45
    regional psychotic symptoms 45-46
    semantic decision task 48, 49
    task performance, SPECT imaging 14
    verbal fluency 47
    word generation and repetition 47-48
    see also brain function

cerebral blood flow (CBF)
    cognitive function 46

Brain Imaging in Schizophrenia